	DATE DUE		

Critical Care

André Picard

CRITICAL CARE

Canadian Nurses Speak for Change

A Phyllis Bruce Book
HarperCollins*PublishersLtd*

Canadian Cataloguing in Publication Data

Picard, André, 1960–
Critical care : Canadian nurses speak for change

"A Phyllis Bruce book."
ISBN 0-00-255726-6

1. Nursing – Canada.
2. Nurses – Canada.
I. Title.

RT6.A1P52 2000   610.73'0971   C00-930094-5

00 01 02 03 04 HC 8 7 6 5 4 3 2 1

Printed and bound in the United States
Set in Sabon

CONTENTS

Part Three: GROWING INTO ADULTHOOD

Part Four: THE ADULT YEARS

Part Five: MENTAL HEALTH

Part Eight: NURSING AND BEYOND

PREFACE

In our society, virtually no one goes through life untouched by nurses. They are there to cradle us at birth, to offer us comfort at death, and to provide care for us at every stage of life in between. Yet nursing has long been not only an invisible profession, but a silent one.

In this book, I have attempted to give nurses more visibility—and a voice. In Canada, three out of four health professionals are nurses, so it is important that we understand the critical role nursing plays in our health system. But, what do nurses *do*? What is this mysterious art called "caring"? *Critical Care* tries to answer these questions by observing the work of nurses in dozens of specialties, in a variety of settings, and by letting nurses themselves tell their stories.

Readers will learn that not only do nurses do a lot—more than most patients ever imagined—they also have a lot to say. What will also become clear is that nursing is more than a profession: it is a social movement, one that has not been given its due. There are ongoing issues that affect nurses—and, by extension, their patients, from all sectors of Canadian society—every day. As nurses face shortages, cutbacks, shift work, and poor working conditions, it is no wonder that they are becoming increasingly politicized, and their patients increasingly worried about the future of health care in Canada.

It is crucial for nurses that they speak up, to protect and defend their important role. But it is doubly important for patients, because nurses are not only their principal caregivers, but also their chief advocates. In the debate over health-care reform, the collective voice of Canada's 263,000 nurses has largely been ignored, often with devastating results.

In many ways, bathing a patient typifies the art of nursing. During this seemingly simple task, a nurse can perform a detailed health assessment: helping a person into the tub can answer questions about mobility; swishing a warm sponge across the skin can detect bed sores; gently cleansing a wound can disclose infection; scrubbing the fingernails can provide important clues about circulation; towelling dry can evaluate balance; and a seemingly innocuous chat can retrieve a detailed medical history and provide insight into a patient's psychological state.

Theoretically, when I began the research for this book, I understood this concept—this notion that simple tasks done well by someone with training and experience can be as valuable as a formal physical examination. But actually seeing nurses at work— giving baths, changing dressings, filling out forms, with an eye to all the other details—is impressive indeed. And, for someone who has struggled to provide care to a loved one, it is humbling.

Critical Care examines nursing throughout the life cycle, beginning with labour and delivery, and closing (almost) with palliative home care; in between, it visits a wide range of nursing specialties. Each of the eight parts offers a brief overview of the health status and the particular concerns of a particular age group. The exceptions are a section devoted to mental-health nursing, which I felt deserved particular emphasis, and a section on nursing outside the clinical setting, which discusses health policy from a nursing perspective.

The individual profiles are not so much portraits of individual women (or men) as profiles of the jobs these individuals do. None of the nurses featured sought a place in the limelight. On the contrary, most agreed to be interviewed only because doing so would raise the profile of their profession and of their particular specialty, not highlight their personal stories. It was not my intention to hold up these particular nurses as heroes or as ideals. In fact, what struck me most forcefully is their ordinariness; at the same time, the stories they tell are fascinating.

I have deliberately adopted some unusual stylistic conventions in this book. For example, I have included no physical descriptions of the principal subjects, and only cursory information about their employers. I chose this approach because, for far too long, more emphasis has been placed on nurses' looks than on their talents as caregivers; as well, I wanted my interview subjects to speak freely. Much of what we read about health care is the opinion of doctors and politicians; this book exclusively expresses the nurses' point of view, whenever possible in their own words.

You will not find any media stereotypes of nurses in *Critical Care*. Instead, you will find team players who know their precise role; caring professionals who know their limits; highly intelligent women and men who learn, and teach, continually; nurses who care deeply for their patients, and carry unbelievable workloads so as not to shortchange them.

There is no mention of specific patients in this book. I was, time and time again, a privileged witness to the very special relationship between nurses and their patients, and I accepted an ethical responsibility to protect their privacy.

I could fill yet another book with praise for nurses from patients. Every time I spoke to patients, or was introduced as an observer, they went out of their way to compliment nurses. The respect and admiration are genuine; the trust nurses earn, well deserved. Yet, when I asked patients what the nurse does for them, the response was often surprised silence. Many said simply, and quite accurately, "She cares for me." But when pressed for details, people could rarely describe more than superficial tasks: "She gives me my chemo drugs"; "She got me ready for surgery"; "She watches the monitors to make sure my baby's okay."

This invisibility is, at once, a blessing and a curse. We don't really give much thought to what nurses do because we know, above all, that they do good. Nurses are, by far, the most trusted professionals in Canada. In the annual "Public Trust Index," a survey conducted by Pollara to gauge which professionals are the most trusted, nurses are always on top, garnering around 97 per cent.

If nurses are so valued by patients, why is the profession not equally valued in our society? Regrettably, while it is rarely stated to be the case, caring is generally regarded as something lesser than medical intervention, and as women's work. There is also an unstated belief that caring and compassion, the hallmarks of a good nurse, can be provided by virtually anyone.

These lingering notions are not only wrong-headed, but also expensive. It used to be that women chose nursing as a career because, for many, it was the most attractive of four choices: nurse, teacher, secretary, housewife. Today, women have many more options, so, if the profession is to attract the best candidates, it must be respected and understood. Virtually every nurse you speak to will say that he or she wants to make a difference. But it is hard to do that in an atmosphere of indifference that often borders on disdain.

Make no mistake about it: nurses are tired of being taken for granted. The most glaring sign is that the profession is not renewing itself. Many second- or third-generation nurses are not urging their daughters and sons to follow in their footsteps. It is projected that, by the year 2011, Canada will face a shortage of 113,000 nurses. Those who are responsible for hiring—the nurse coordinators in institutions and the community, the hospital vice-presidents, the administrators of regional health-care boards and home-care agencies—know there is already a crisis, and that it intensifies with each passing month.

Several factors are fuelling this crisis. The number of places in nursing schools is clearly inadequate. Experienced nurses are fleeing the profession, driven away by chronic overwork, inadequate pay, and terrible working conditions. Young nurses are not being attracted to the profession in sufficient numbers. And why should they be?

Nursing is hard—physically demanding and mentally exhausting, particularly when shift work is required. Nurses have borne the brunt of financial cutbacks in the health-care system, many of them having gone a decade without a raise. Most have been denied long-overdue pay-equity adjustments. Meanwhile, the workload increases unrelentingly as the population ages, health-care staffing declines, and more and more tasks are off-loaded onto nurses.

It's not that starting wages are bad—they range from an hourly rate of $15.10 in Newfoundland, to $20.98 in British Columbia—but the maximum wages of nurses are disgracefully low—about $27 an hour for a unionized hospital nurse. A nurse with thirty years' experience at the bedside makes about the same as someone with ten years' worth. Performance bonuses are unheard of in the profession. Nurse-researchers, who have played a key role in some major drug breakthroughs, earn significantly less than hospital nurses. Many community nurses are paid poverty-level wages. In the Maritime provinces, some home-care nurses earn only $11 an hour—less than zookeepers.

There have been many nurses on the picket lines of late. They are not out there principally because of money concerns, but because of their work conditions. Personnel shortages have meant that some nurses have gone years without a holiday. They get a lot of overtime, but they get burned out. Tens of thousands of part-time nurses (whose status confers no benefits, no paid holidays, no pension) work full-time hours.

The result? Nurses take 50 per cent more sick days than the average worker. They have above-average drug- and alcohol-abuse rates. Their stress levels are through the roof. The on-the-job hazards are many: needle sticks and the blood-borne pathogens they carry, violent patients, chemicals ranging from disinfectants to laser plume (the smoke released during surgery), not to mention back injuries,* which afflict four in ten nurses. Yet, one would be hard-pressed to name a single health-care institution

---

* The occupational-health standard is that a worker should not lift a weight of more than 17 kilograms, but nurses routinely lift many times that weight when moving patients. They are also on their feet for most of their twelve-hour shifts.

in the country that has an occupational-health nurse on staff to take care of its own workers.

The nurses you will meet in *Critical Care* work in a variety of settings, in various parts of the country, and in numerous specialties. They do not represent a perfect cross-section of the profession today, as 62 per cent of nurses work in hospitals, another 10 per cent in nursing homes, and only 6 per cent in community health (see chart, page 247, for 1996 statisctics). But the specialties visited here do reflect the broad range of the profession.

Because I wanted this book to be forward-looking, I have included a disproportionate number of community-health nurses. In fact, if there is a bias in this book, it is towards prevention. This is a grossly neglected field, but one that, with proper investment, can bring financial stability to our universal health-care system. It is also an area in which nurses excel, and have been blazing a trail for 350 years.

A theme that runs throughout *Critical Care* is the importance of investing not only in good, solid medical care, but also in public health (and public-health nurses) to create a system that provides humane treatment for illness, and promotes wellness—a concept that has been marginalized and undervalued, much as nurses have been.

Many of the nurses I interviewed were researchers—a role that has never been adequately acknowledged. Many were often the best people to describe, clearly and succinctly, what nurses *do*, which is the focus of this book.

Almost 80 per cent of nurses currently practising in Canada are diploma-prepared, meaning that they trained in a hospital or graduated from a community-college program. All of those featured in *Critical Care* are registered nurses, with either a Bachelor of Nursing or a Bachelor of Science degree, though many got their degrees after many years of working in the field. Many of the nurses interviewed have a master's degree, and more than a few have a doctorate. Education, as well as being mandatory—in five provinces, a registered nurse now needs a minimum of a bachelor's degree—is also the route to specialized jobs. Several of the nurses featured are nurse-practitioners, performing functions that were once the exclusive domain of physicians.

During my research, I was struck at how quickly specialization is becoming the norm. A number of nursing specialties already have their own accreditation process. But specialization brings its own problems, chief among them nurses' fear that they will become more distanced from their patients, as physicians have over the years. Nurses also have to be careful that, in the rush to specialize, they not be relegated to the role of junior doctors, be assigned the drudgery instead of being permitted to use their unique talents.

Because of shortages, nurses have much opportunity for movement within the profession, not only from hospitals to the community, but from one specialty to another. However, the details of what is involved in a particular type of specialty nursing are as obscure to nurses in any other specialty as they are to the general public. Trauma nurses with highly specialized training, for example, do not always understand the challenges faced by nurses practising at a remote nursing station; the daily reality of pediatric-AIDS nurses in a hospital setting is dramatically different from that of street nurses working with AIDS patients, even though they may be only blocks apart geographically; the nurse offering chronic care does work that is entirely different from that of a nurse who does palliative care. There is no longer a "typical" nurse.

During my years as a journalist, I have met nurses in every imaginable setting: in corporate boardrooms, in war zones, at political rallies, and in shanty-towns. Some of those nurses are featured in Part Eight: "Nursing and Beyond." While some of them no longer do "hands-on" nursing, every one of them says that, no matter how long ago you stopped wearing scrubs, you never stop being a nurse. Many stress that the traits required to be a good nurse—the ability to listen, to digest information quickly, to analyse, to prioritize, and to act decisively—serve them well, particularly in business.

This book has been a personal as well as a professional journey for me. I have written about health care for many years, but I was surprised at how little I knew about what nurses do. Many of us in the so-called sandwich generation start to care about nursing when we have children, and when our parents' health declines. I felt there was a knowledge gap that needed to be filled.

As a journalist and public-policy writer, I have followed the tainted-blood tragedy for almost a decade. During that time, I met hundreds of victims, many of them very bitter. Many of the infected hemophiliacs had, as children, attended clinics where the products were injected by nurses; many of the transfusion patients remember quite clearly the assurances of nurses that the products they were getting were safe. (Nurses, like consumers, were recipients of grossly irresponsible misinformation.) But, in all that time, I never heard a word said against a nurse.

That intrigued me, and doubly so because both of my parents had chronic illnesses—my late father, Alzheimer's, and my mother, chronic obstructive pulmonary disorder—that required much nursing care, in the hospital, the community, and a nursing home. Nurses saved my mom's life. I know. I was there. Nurses cared for my father, feeding him, bathing him, and changing him when he lost the ability to do so himself. Just as important, nurses were there to ensure the quality of his death.

This book is, above all, for them.

I hope *Critical Care* will promote greater public respect for nursing. And I hope this book will remind nurses themselves that, after years of being ignored, what they do is still very special, and that there are many opportunities in this vast profession called nursing.

As a 90-year-old man with colon cancer said to me in Victoria: "You only need to be a patient one time to know the value of nursing."

A NURSING PIONEER

Helen Mussallem graduated from the nursing school at Vancouver General Hospital in 1937. She recalls that the class was remarkable for two reasons: "We were the first students to be taught to take blood pressure. That was considered high-tech at the time, if you can imagine. We were also the first class to get clinical training." But the greatest claim to fame of the class of '37 is Mussallem herself, a trailblazer who helped to fundamentally reshape Canada's health-care system and, along the way, became a living legend. Her fascinating career is a microcosm of the evolution of modern nursing, and she remains a powerful influence today.

Nursing began in Canada more than three centuries ago, when Marie Hubou established "missions of healing and mercy" with the help of colonial nuns. The Nursing Sisters of Dieppe opened the country's first hospital, Hôtel-Dieu Montreal. Subsequently, Marguerite Bourgeoys and Marguerite d'Youville, of the Congregation of the Sisters of Charity of the Hôpital Général of Montreal (Grey Nuns), founded more than 100 hospitals in Upper and Lower Canada. The Victorian Order of Nurses began its work in 1897, firmly establishing nurses in the community and as purveyors of health promotion. Émilie Tavernier-Gamelin, founder of the Daughters of Charity, inspired the creation of numerous hospitals in Canada and the U.S. in the late nineteenth century.

During the twentieth century, nurses continued their key role in the community. In the 1920s, the Red Cross built more than 100 outpost hospitals in rural Canada, and established life-saving vaccination programs. During the Depression, nurses concerned themselves with social ills such as child malnutrition, in addition to providing medical care, and helping create the foundation for the public-health system that would emerge later out of Prairie populism.

During the Second World War, nurses like Helen Mussallem played an invaluable role. A surgical nurse, she joined the No. 19 Royal Canadian Army Medical Corps as a lieutenant and, after a short stint training soldiers to become medical technicians, went overseas to minister to the sick and wounded at the front. Nurses in battlefield hospitals were responsible for triage, doing minor medical operations such as stitching and suturing, and assisting surgeons. "It was very, very basic. Our job was to patch the soldiers up enough to get them back to Canada alive," Mussallem says.

The war gave her a very different taste of nursing. Unlike their civilian counterparts, army nurses had broad responsibilities and were quite respected. Mussallem recalls a soldier coming in with a badly damaged leg, a wound infested with maggots. Limbs in such poor condition were routinely amputated, but in this instance the surgeon asked the nurse her opinion. "I said: 'Sir, the boy told me that if you cut off his leg, he will die.' " The doctor put away the surgical saw, and had her clean the wound and place the leg in a cast. "I was so thrilled to be a respected part of the team," she says. But not as thrilled as she was when, long after, she was disembarking from a ship after the war and heard a man yelling, "Sister, Sister, Sister." The soldier, still on crutches, embraced her and said: "Sister, I still have two legs. Thank you."

After the war, Mussallem used her veteran's points* to study at McGill University, beginning a lifelong love of and dedication to education. The Bachelor of Nursing (BN) was quite special then; there were only twelve women in the class and, even during their studies, bachelor's students taught those in the certificate program. Mussallem returned to Vancouver General for a decade, holding a

---

* Veterans were awarded points, essentially government credits, that could be used for subsidized education or to purchase low-cost land.

variety of management and teaching positions. During that period, she continued studying, getting a teaching certificate at the University of Washington and a master's degree at Columbia University in New York. (She was able to do this in part because her father, a wealthy businessman and well-known municipal politician in British Columbia, provided financial support.)

In 1957, however, she accepted a contract with the Canadian Nurses Association (CNA) that would change not only her career, but the nursing profession itself. There were, at the time, no set standards for teaching or clinical practice, so Mussallem set out to evaluate the state of nursing education. She travelled more than 90,000 kilometres, interviewing 2,000 nurses and dissecting the work of twenty-five nursing schools around the country.

Her 1957 report, *Spotlight on Nursing Education in Canada*, was a bombshell. In it, she wrote that education standards were disgraceful, that students were little more than indentured labourers. (Virtually all training was done by hospitals, who forced the nurses to live in residences and guaranteed themselves a cheap workforce.) The result, she concluded, was unacceptably substandard care at many institutions. "There was fire coming out of the end of my pen when I was writing that report. I couldn't believe there were so many poor schools of nursing, that only one in four was up to standard," Mussallem recalls. The report infuriated hospital administrators and gave a big boost to university programs. It also launched the unionization movement among nurses; shortly after the report was released, nurses at her alma mater in Vancouver went on strike—the first time in Canada that nurses walked a picket line.

Mussallem extended her contract to oversee an implementation committee. "People say that report was a landmark, but they give me too much credit. The credit has to go to the head nurses and nursing supervisors who fought with their hospital administrators to get the recommendations implemented, to forever change the way nurses are educated," she says. In her report, she noted that no library in Canada had holdings of reference material oriented to nursing. The Canadian Nurses Association established such a resource and, many years later, it was, fittingly, named the Helen K. Mussallem Library.

While working on education reform, Mussallem accepted another life-altering contract. She agreed to serve, for four months, as the executive director of the Canadian Nurses Association, a position she ended up holding until 1981. That period was perhaps the most exciting ever in Canadian health care, from the creation of the building blocks of medicare through to the tumultuous period of its consolidation as a national program under what ultimately became the Canada Health Act. "Medicare changed the profession and the country dramatically," Mussallem says. During her tenure, the number of nurses and university-based training programs for nurses soared, and nursing specialties were initiated.

In her 1963 CNA submission to the Royal Commission on Health Care, titled "Putting the Health Back into Health Care," she called for a shift to community care, and a massive investment in preventive medicine, not to mention a call for all doctors to be salaried; these recommendations were ignored by Mr. Justice Emmett Hall, but, almost forty years later, are being touted as the remedies for an ailing health-care system.

Mussallem wrote another groundbreaking report in 1969, titled *The Changing Role of the Nurse.* Laid up after a serious back injury, she envisaged the idea of community-based health clinics that would be run by nurses, and established in shopping malls, nursing homes, churches, and other places people congregate. "The idea was to have nursing posts as community institutions, and every citizen would report to the nurse, whether sick or well. They would be the gatekeepers to the health system," Mussallem recalls. Several years later, Quebec would establish such a network, called Centre local de services communautaires (CLSCs), but, fearing political backlash, the province did not stop funding family practices, thereby creating a redundancy. Though she was out there preaching the gospel of preventive medicine and community nursing, virtually everyone blissfully ignored it—with predictable results.

Throughout the 1970s, the role of nurses changed substantially, as did the role of women in society. The director of nursing moved up in the hospital hierarchy; community-health projects sprang up all over, and so did independent nurse-practitioners. Mussallem was at the forefront of many of these movements, and taking on other challenges as well—some of them, such as the battle for reproductive choice, quite controversial. As a nurse who had witnessed abortions performed in kitchens on women who were in dire economic straits and unable to pay for health care, she was unflinching in her views and compelling in her arguments. "I fought my entire life for nursing. I was always in a scrap over something, and I didn't lose very often," Mussallem says. Her accomplishments in the field are unique; she was the first nurse in Canada to get a doctorate.

After her "retirement" at age 66, Mussallem became a roving health ambassador, promoting nursing and education in more than forty countries and publishing dozens of scholarly articles. (In many countries, she did exactly what she had done in Canada earlier, dissecting the nursing-education programs and helping to rebuild them to rigorous standards.)

She also played an important backroom role in the production of one of the Canada's most important pieces of legislation, the Canada Health Act. In the early 1980s, as today, health-care budgets were soaring, services varied greatly from province to province, new technologies were springing up daily, and there was much talk of following the United States down the path to privatization. In response, Health Minister Monique Bégin produced 1984 legislation that enshrined free, universal health care—though, at the last minute, she backed down from the position Mussallem held: that universality should apply not only to physician and hospital services, but also to community-based programs such as nurse-staffed clinics and home care.

In the meantime, Mussallem's honours kept piling up. She was named Companion of the Order of Canada. The Royal College of Nurses of the United Kingdom described Mussallem as "Canada's most distinguished nurse of her time and generation." St. John Ambulance invested her with a Dame of Grace, its highest grade. The International Red Cross awarded her with the Florence Nightingale Medal. She also received honorary degrees from six universities.

Mussallem says modestly that many of these honours were intended for, and rightfully belong to, Canada's health-care system and the nurses who toil daily to deliver quality, universal, and free health care. "I lived in an era when patients died because they didn't have the money to pay for medical services, and I'm proud to say I played a part in ending that injustice, in creating a system for everyone. It's said quite often, but I don't think Canadians truly appreciate what they have. Medicare was the best thing that ever happened to this nation; it defines us as caring and compassionate people," she stresses. "And no one contributes more to the health of Canadians than nurses."

Part One
THE EARLY YEARS

In the Nurse's Arms

The number one reason for hospital admission in Canada is child-birth. Each of the 400,000 children born annually will come into contact with a nurse in his or her early years, and likely repeatedly, for everything from vaccinations to heart conditions.

The first person a newborn baby sees is usually a nurse or a midwife (most of whom are former nurses). The vast majority of babies will be healthy, but infancy is nonetheless a tumultuous time. Anxious parents make many trips to emergency rooms and clinics, and the result is that the rate of hospitalization for infants is the highest for any age group.

One in three babies will spend time in hospital during the first year of life. The majority suffer from perinatal conditions such as low birth weight (the leading cause of death of newborns), respiratory diseases, and birth defects. Infants with underdeveloped immune systems, particularly those who are not breast-fed, fall prey to viruses and bacteria. They are also at high risk for injury, notably from suffocation.

As children grow, their motor skills develop more quickly than their reasoning skills, putting them at high risk for injury. Almost half of all deaths among Canada's 1.8 million preschoolers are the result of injuries, from falls and motor-vehicle accidents. And for every child killed, there are seventy-five who will have serious injuries—many resulting in permanent disability—that require hospital care.

But the biggest threat to the health of Canadian children is probably poverty. Mothers who are poor eat badly. Many, for a variety of social reasons, smoke. The result is low-birth-weight babies.

In Montreal, a group of public-health nurses developed a program called "oeufs-lait-oranges" (OLO). When a pregnant woman walks into a CLSC (Centre local de services communautaires) in the city's poorest neighbourhoods, she is sent directly to a nurse and given an unusual prescription—eggs, milk, and oranges. Innovative programs such as OLO can have a lifelong influence on children, and a dramatic financial impact on the health-care system, but they remain an anomaly.

An estimated 1.2 million children in the "best country on Earth" live below the poverty line. Shocking disparities exist among children, based on parental income, marital status, ethnic background, and physical ability. Being poor means a child is many times more likely to face ill health, a reality the Canadian Institute of Child Health calls a "dark smear on the integrity of our society."

While prevention continues to get short shrift, we are fortunate that considerable money has been invested in technology and in specialists to save children's lives. Babies born months premature and weighing less than half a kilogram now can be kept alive, thanks to sophisticated equipment and knowledge gained over the years. Surgery can now be done not only on tiny newborns, but in vitro. It is often forgotten that much of the knowledge that led to these techniques came from nurses, who care for premature babies around the clock.

In Part One, you will meet nurses who work with the youngest and most vulnerable members of our society, beginning with labour and delivery nurse Debbie Gauthier. Toiling in Regina, the birthplace of medicare, she offers insight on the impact of cutbacks on nurses and their patients—in particular, on birthing mothers.

Neonatal nurse Kathy Hamelin works with the fragile creatures we affectionately call "preemies." (There are more than 22,000 low-birth-weight babies born in Canada annually.) Nowhere is the dichotomy of pediatric nursing more obvious than in her workplace. Many of the mothers with high-risk births at Winnipeg Health Sciences Centre are desperately poor Native women. They are surrounded by millions of dollars' worth of medical machinery, yet what they need more than anything is to give up smoking and to relearn the importance of breast-feeding. Hamelin is also an international expert on premature twins, and an example of the growing role of nurse-researcher. Her research on co-bedding—which examined anecdotal evidence presented by nurses and parents that twins who sleep together breathe easier—has changed practices around the world.

Another nursing trailblazer who works with newborns is Penny Triggs. A flight nurse, she spirits mothers with high-risk pregnancies and children with health problems (largely respiratory problems) out of Nunavut, a massive territory with no hospitals and virtually no doctors. Triggs has not only provided much hands-on care over the years, but helped to shape and professionalize the specialty known as "medical evacuation."

Hospital admissions of children have fallen by half during the past decade, but the work of nurses has not diminished. Cases today are more acute and complex, and parents are more demanding health-care consumers. Pediatrics nurse Claire Sheinman Cowan heads a multidisciplinary team at St. Joseph's Health Centre. At the west-end Toronto hospital, she is trying to create programs that not only will provide care to children who are sick and injured, but will supply a place where parents can go to seek advice on all kinds of health and disease-prevention issues.

Paula Robeson is undertaking a similar task, but in a different venue. A nurse and policy analyst at the Canadian Institute of Child Health, she works in a dreary west-end Ottawa office tower, but has one of the most important jobs in health care today: she is trying to shape the spending priorities of governments, emphasizing the importance of spending on the early years to avoid lifelong health problems and costs.

Less than 4 per cent of Canada's $86-billion health budget is spent on prevention. As such, ours is not a health system, but a disease-treatment system, one that is financially untenable over the long term. Nurses across the country are at the forefront of trying to save the medicare system by reinventing it, by shifting the focus to prevention.

Here, more than anywhere else, lies the unrealized potential of nursing. Knowledge—not medicine—is what makes people healthy. Nurses are not only caregivers, but teachers. By instilling healthy habits in expectant mothers, their children, and their families, they can change lives dramatically.

The Labours of Delivery—Debbie Gauthier

When Debbie Gauthier began working as a labour and delivery nurse in 1975, expectant mothers were prepared for the birth as they would be for surgery. They were given a hospital gown and an enema, had their pubic hair shaved, and were forbidden to shower or eat. When the contractions were at short, regular intervals, the mother-to-be was rolled down the hall to a sterile operating room, sometimes under anaesthetic and often after having received drugs to speed up the labour. There, the woman's feet were placed in stirrups, and nurses and doctors, clad in masks and gowns, delivered the baby, using an array of tools such as forceps and vacuum extractors. Mother and baby were separated almost immediately, and despatched to separate recovery rooms.

The love affair with technology and institutional process that gripped the health-care system in the 1960s and 1970s not only was alienating to patients, but also stood in the way of nurses doing what they did best—providing care on a one-to-one basis.

Since then, the birthing process in Canadian hospitals has changed dramatically, thanks to a combination of consumer revolt and nursing advocacy. Many hospitals have constructed homey birthing facilities, and the interventionist medical approach has been scaled back considerably. In fact, many of the changes that have occurred in the health-care system during the past generation, notably the voice now accorded patients, had their genesis in obstetrics.

Gauthier, who in her time at Regina General Hospital has participated in thousands of deliveries, was all too happy to cast off the mask and spend time with a labouring mother who was in bed rather than strapped to a surgical gurney. Herself a mother, she knew first-hand how cold and frustrating a hospital birth could be. She set out to alter the rules.

Today, Gauthier says, the mix of technology and old-fashioned caring is much more even. Advances such as ultrasound and electronic fetal monitors allow for better screening and fewer unpleasant surprises, and staff reductions have meant that nurses are now the prime caregivers during most of the birthing process.

While much nursing in an institutional setting is task-oriented, a good labour and delivery-room nurse takes a patient-centred approach. Gauthier sees her principal role as ensuring that women get the kind of delivery they want (some want an all-natural birth, while others are preoccupied with pain relief), with as few complications as possible. "When you do this job, you soon realize that it's a once-in-a-lifetime experience for each patient. They want to be treated like their delivery is the most important one that has ever been done, and my job is to try and make them feel that way," Gauthier says. A large part of doing this job well is having a knack for knowing what a patient will need next, because "you can never do anything fast enough for a labouring woman. When they want something, they want it *now*," Gauthier says with a knowing smile.

Research has shown that obstetrics patients who have someone sitting with them have much easier deliveries, and those who receive coaching do better still. Ideally, then, labour and delivery nurses try to provide one-on-one care (though two or three patients at a time is now the norm) and balance that constant vigilance with unobtrusiveness. A nurse who comes in for a quiet chat is usually checking the fetal monitor and assessing a woman's demeanour for early signs of potentially grave problems such as preeclampsia.

Deliveries at a hospital such as Regina General, which handles most of the high-risk births in the province, are particularly

labour-intensive. Insulin-dependent diabetics, women with preg-
nancy-induced hypertension, multiple births, and severely premature labours need constant attention.

A delivery room is also unpredictable: a labouring mother—or
two, three, or four—can walk through the door at any time and,
because labour varies greatly from one woman to the next, the
delivery can be minutes or many hours away. Contrary to popular belief, Gauthier says, all babies are not born in the middle of
the night. Elective Caesareans—many of them necessary because
of high-risk factors—are performed during the day.

At the beginning of a shift, which runs from 7:30 A.M. to 8:00
P.M., or from 7:30 P.M. to 8:00 A.M., nurses receive reports on all
the patients present and those who are scheduled to be admitted.
When they are assigned principal responsibility for a patient, they
get a more detailed report from the nurse they are relieving. The new
nurse reads the chart and does a reassessment of her own. From that
point on, care depends on the needs of the patient. Some just want
to talk; others want a tub bath or pain relief. At the hospital, use of
fetal monitors is routine, and they are checked every five to fifteen
minutes. When labour is active, nurses rarely leave the room.

An increasingly important and time-consuming role for nurses
is monitoring and controlling the comings and goings of other
family members. Having a partner, parent, or doula* present for
a birth is now almost routine, but relatives can sometimes be as
much work as the mother, and more unpredictable. "We lose most
husbands during the epidural insertion.† But you get pretty good
at knowing when they're going to faint, so not many hit the floor,"
Gauthier jokes.

Obstetricians check in with patients occasionally—generally,
with a normal labour, they are not called until the baby's head is
visible—but nurses are there through every stage of the process,

---

* "Doula" is a Greek word for an experienced woman who helps other women,
in this case a birth companion or labour assistant.
† To provide pain relief, a tube is inserted into the labouring mother's back and
anaesthetic is introduced into the space around the spinal cord.

whether the labour is easy and lasts one hour or is a gruelling overnighter. When the birth is very fast, a nurse does the delivery without a physician present. Gauthier does about four each month, and considers it routine.

What troubles her, however, is that doctors are not always available when a nurse spots a potential problem. While she is an advocate for midwifery, Gauthier does not believe nurses should be delivering every baby, particularly not high-risk cases. "Most of the physicians we work with are wonderful. When there is a problem, they earn every penny they get," she says. What labour and delivery-room nurses resent is when a doctor comes in at the end of a long labour and starts coaching or insisting on procedures a woman is not comfortable with, rather than trusting the relationship that has developed between the woman and the nurse. "The good ones come in and quietly deliver the baby. They show their confidence in the nursing staff by playing their role on the team instead of trying to take over," she says.

With a quarter-century of experience in the delivery room, Debbie Gauthier is not that unusual. Obstetrics nurses, unlike those in many other specialties, tend to stay their entire careers. Bringing children into the world, and making the experience a little more pleasant and memorable for mothers and fathers alike, is one of the most rewarding jobs in medicine.

But there are nights nurses dread. "What I hate is when you're on the night shift and it's a little too quiet until after midnight, and then the bus comes in," Gauthier says, using the delivery-room parlance for an influx of patients. While three or four labouring mothers is typical for a shift at Regina General, there have been nights when the number reaches a dozen, far above capacity. Worse yet is a shift that sees a half-dozen cases, each one of them with complications.

In an area of nursing where it is easy to fill vacancies, staff shortages hit home all the same. Most hospitals—and obstetrics departments, in particular—used to have huge float pools of help and could call in staff at short notice. Today, such pools are virtually non-existent, and regular staff are often called in to work overtime.

Gauthier will get an average of three overtime shifts per month (with the calls invariably coming in the middle of the night) on top of her dozen regular twelve-hour-plus workdays. That schedule takes a toll, particularly on the veteran nurses who are the core obstetrics group.

Another downside of working in labour and delivery is the emotional toll it can take. In high-risk centres, babies die, and mothers do too. "There are a minority of cases that are awful ones—where you lose the baby or the mother—but the heartbreak stays with you for years. This is a job where you have a lot of sleepless nights because sometimes, when you close your eyes, you just relive some cases," Gauthier says sadly.

Yet the greatest strain in her daily work comes from the lack of upgrading of facilities, which she blames on spending cutbacks. Despite the philosophical changes that have taken place, the labour and delivery unit at Regina General looks very much as it did when birthing mothers were herded through like cattle. The rooms do not have private bathrooms; there are only two tubs on a ward with eight birthing rooms; the rooms are so small that having partners present interferes with the work of doctors and nurses; the beds are not only old, but in sorry condition (limiting the variety of delivery positions); there is only one operating room; and the recovery unit is a five-bed ward with no privacy. These surroundings don't inspire confidence.

Throughout the medical system, specialization is increasing, which generally aids patients, but often the priorities for resource allocation are wrong. In birthing, for example, most cases require only minimal medical intervention, and the investment should be in comfort for the patients. At the same time, those who do require highly specialized medical care see too much attention diverted to routine cases that could be handled by midwives or nurses alone.

There have been dramatic and welcome changes in labour and delivery. Women have achieved greater comfort and more choice. But the options available to them—and the ability of nurses to provide the kind of care they want and need—are still inadequate.

A Celebration of Life—Kathy Hamelin

The leading cause of infant mortality in Canada is prematurity. Infants born well before term have lungs so underdeveloped that breathing is difficult. Of the 400,000 children born each year in Canada, about 1,200 die at birth because of respiratory problems and low birth weight. Yet medical researchers do not really know why babies are born so early that their lives are endangered. Until enough is known to develop methods of prevention, there is only treatment, and much of that is provided by nurses.

There are few medical fields in which progress has been as spectacular as it has been in premature birth. The rate of perinatal and neonatal deaths has fallen from 32.5 per 1,000 in 1971 to 12.3 per 1,000 in 1990. Babies born at twenty-four weeks are now viable, and half survive; at thirty weeks, birth is almost routine (even though a full term is about forty weeks). While technology has played a significant part in these gains, much of the improvement in survival rates is due to the observations of nurses, who care for the precarious newborns around the clock. These tiny infants— some so small that a washcloth serves as a receiving blanket—face enormous health challenges.

Until less than a decade ago, preemies were snatched from their mothers and whisked away to an incubator and a barrage of technology. It could be months before parents were allowed to hold their child, and, then, visiting hours were limited. More often than not, the babies did not survive.

Today, getting babies to bond and to breast-feed is considered almost as important to them as healthy breathing apparatus. "We used to think that families were in the way, but today we realize they are essential to survival," says Kathy Hamelin, a neonatal clinical nurse-specialist at Women's Hospital, of the Winnipeg Health Sciences Centre. "When you think about it, if these babies are only half-done, then their moms are only half-done with the pregnancy too. We realize now that family is probably even more important to the preemie than to the full-term baby. We have totally changed our nursing practice to reflect that realization."

Hamelin, one of the country's foremost researchers in neonatology, was an early proponent of the kangaroo method, whereby underdeveloped newborns are cuddled against the bare skin of a parent as if they were in the womb. So, premature babies weighing as little as 900 grams and fitting easily in the palm of the hand, once considered too fragile to touch, now spend upwards of eight hours daily clinging to their mother. All parents have around-the-clock access to their babies, and many live on-site.

"I learned more from the fifty moms in the first kangaroo-care trial than I learned in twenty years of nursing. What they told us is that hospitals have to support mothers to become mothers in spite of the technology. That, to me, is what neonatal nursing is all about," she says.

Hamelin also advocates early breast-feeding, an approach that was, until recently, considered folly. Now, babies born at thirty weeks are often at the breast the same day. And 85 per cent of pre-term mothers at Women's Hospital go home breast-feeding.

For a nurse to be a clinical researcher is still unusual, but it is an essential means of improving health care. Nurses are there, at the bedside, twenty-four hours a day, and they accumulate tremendous knowledge. They can tap into that knowledge to validate what they observed and update clinical practice. For example, preemies used to be routinely laid on their stomachs, because that position facilitated breathing. But, after months of being face down, many could not even move their hands to their face, leading to all sorts of developmental delays. Similarly, research found that preemies who had no contact with their parents for months would grow up to become victims of abuse in disproportionately large numbers.

At any one time, Hamelin will have a handful of research projects on the go. An essential element is recruiting parents, and that process requires that the researcher offer education. Hamelin is a lactation consultant, teaches cardiopulmonary resuscitation for babies, and provides other practical assistance for parents, such as finding car seats suitable for tiny preemies.

The research for which Hamelin is making her mark, the co-bedding of twins, is groundbreaking. (She stresses repeatedly, however, that research is a team effort.) Many premature children are part of multiple births, but traditionally they were kept apart, owing to the risks of infection. However, mothers found that premature twins kept apart had numerous breathing crises and grew up to be extremely difficult to parent. Mothers who had their children sleep together reported that they were far more settled and calm, and that, by snuggling together, they had lower oxygen demands; they also kept to the same schedule, which is a tremendous benefit to beleaguered parents.

Hamelin has been involved in testing a number of drugs that boost the production of breast milk (these drugs, initially used to treat digestive problems, were found to double the milk supply overnight), and others to treat the ailments that impede feeding. She rails against the illogic of a health-care system that discourages mothers of babies with thrush from breast-feeding because the treatment is a $300 prescription when, over time, those "savings" will cost the system dearly. "If you look at the pediatric hospitals in this country, an overwhelming number of the patients are children who were formula-fed babies. So, it's worth making a lot of effort to assist in breast-feeding," she says.

An increasingly large portion of Hamelin's work is outside the hospital, mainly in Winnipeg's aboriginal community. Women's Hospital has created a breast-feeding clinic that provides help to more than 100 new mothers each month, and a telephone hotline that fields hundreds of calls. It has also launched a peer-counselling project to encourage aboriginal moms, the vast majority of whom opt for formula, to breast-feed.

Hamelin's research has led her to become an activist, notably in opposing marketing efforts by infant-formula companies, and taking her concerns to the hospital's board of directors. While the battle has not been entirely successful, Hamelin's advocacy has ensured that at least part of the money—and the hospital has received more than $1 million from one manufacturer alone,

Mead Johnson—gets rerouted back to lactation research.

An experienced and outspoken practitioner, Hamelin does not always see eye to eye with her physician colleagues, and that is particularly true when it comes to promoting breast-feeding. "Lots of them really have a long way to go. They just don't get any education about the benefits of breast-feeding. But nurses tend to see it as a fundamental health-promotion practice," she says. The difference, Hamelin adds, is philosophical: "Neonatal doctors talk about medical issues. I talk about family issues." Ideally, these approaches should be complementary, and she loves her work because, at Women's Hospital, they tend to be.

Like many nurses, Hamelin wears a number of hats. Aside from her research and lactation consulting, she teaches at the University of Manitoba faculty of nursing and is involved in "far too many committee meetings," both within the hospital and with community groups. But the part of her work she truly relishes is that of educator. She teaches staff to ensure that nurses are kept current on the latest clinical developments, and to provide feedback and get new ideas on research.

Though her job is multifaceted, the questions and concerns of high-risk expectant mothers always come first. Hamelin will drop everything to provide a tour to an anxious parent or to offer a shoulder to cry on to a family that has lost a baby. Preparing a family for the arrival of a preemie means helping them to understand the reality of a 1-kilogram baby without scaring them. And counselling grieving parents amidst some of the most sophisticated and expensive medical technology in the world is an equally delicate balancing act.

While Hamelin never discusses her own experience when she speaks to families, it underlies her drive and dedication. Hamelin herself had three high-risk pregnancies, and gave birth to three premature children. Two of them, Mark and Erin, are healthy adults. But her first son, Michael, died shortly after birth in 1972.

"I can still remember the words of the pediatrician. He said: 'Forget it, you can have another.' It was so callous," Hamelin recalls quietly. "I was an employee of the hospital. I was a baby nurse at the time, and that's how I was treated. My baby died on the unit I worked on." As was the practice at the time, she was not allowed to hold her baby. The child was buried, and the hospital refused to tell the parents where. The loss of a premature child was considered a medical failure, and it was supposed to be forgotten immediately, the feelings of parents be damned.

Hamelin left neonatal nursing for a while after that, unable to stomach the sight of a dead child, and turned to teaching and research. But she came back, determined to change the system. Today, when a child dies, parents get time alone with their loved one. Many hospitals also provide a photo of the baby—and it is the job of a nurse to take the picture that will serve as a lasting memory. Women's Hospital also has an annual remembrance service, and a monthly support group.

The treatment of the surviving babies has changed too. The nursery is now dimly lit (many preemies used to be blinded by the bright lights). The rooms full of state-of-the-art equipment are enlivened by bright colours and there are handwritten signs around reading: "S-h-h-h, baby sleeping." (Interestingly, the nursery received funding for an expensive refurbishment after the grandson of a prominent politician was born at the hospital.) Neonatal nurses now take the view that cuddling is sometimes as important as monitoring the oxygen level, that developing the mother–child bond is well worth the slight risk of infection, that emotional care of the parents can be as important as physical care of the baby. Machines cannot replace the care nurses provide, only complement it.

As medical technologies improve and health-care practices evolve, fewer high-risk mothers will have to endure the heart-breaking loss of a child, as Hamelin did years ago, in some part because of the care she and her collegues have provided. While she does not have a photo of her son Michael, she does have in her office a large bulletin board entitled "Wall of Fame," a celebration of the many premature babies that beat the odds and not only survived, but thrived—a celebration of good nursing.

Dreams Take Flight — Penny Triggs

It is -40°C, and a storm is heading in. Your patient, a young child in respiratory distress, has just been transported across town at breakneck speed on a snowmobile. Staff at the nursing station have done their best to stabilize the girl. There are a dozen more children with similar symptoms, but the child has had a series of health problems since being born prematurely earlier in the year. Your job is to get the baby on a plane in Rankin Inlet and deliver her to Winnipeg Health Sciences Centre.

Welcome to a typical day in the life of a medical evacuation nurse in Nunavut. In Canada's newest territory, nurses battle the elements and geography to provide health care, and the closest doctors and hospitals are hundreds of kilometres away, by air. It is a frontier, where they tackle traumas, the epidemics of disease, the high-risk births, along with all the aches and pains of daily living, with equal alacrity.

"Nurses are lifesavers in northern communities, and medevac is their lifeline to the outside world," says Penny Triggs, vice-president of air medical operations at Keewatin Air Ltd., a private company that operates an air-ambulance service on contract for the Nunavut government. Its services are invaluable. Having nomadic populations settle into villages, often in sub-par housing, has had dramatic public-health consequences. There are only 8,000 people in all of Nunavut, and about 400 are flown out for emergency medical treatment each year. The vast majority are children.

Triggs, an experienced intensive-care nurse with more than a decade under her belt as a flight nurse, splits her time between Winnipeg headquarters and Rankin Inlet. She is the details person. When the pager goes off, she takes the call, prepares the medical equipment, lines up flight approval, rounds up a medical and flight crew and dispatches them, and starts preparing for arrival. "When the call comes from a nurse, they're not booking a flight for next week, they want it now—or sooner," she says. The goal is to have the patient airborne within thirty minutes.

The most important part of the job is probably the most mundane: the initial phone call. "You have to get a maximum amount of information about the patient in a minimum of time. The more you know—the vital signs, the medical history, where they are—the more you can plan, and the more you can plan, the smoother the transfer," she notes.

Keewatin's nurses work closely with those in northern outposts. In fact, the company rotates its staff out of the Arctic—one month in, one month off. It is a demanding lifestyle, but they get paid the equivalent of the annual salary of an emergency-room nurse, while working for only six months. The company also provides free housing in Rankin Inlet. During their down time, many nurses travel and study, but many stay and work in isolated nursing stations. Like outpost nurses, flight nurses have protocols that allow them to perform procedures that hospital nurses cannot; they can do defibrilation and airway management, insert needles into bone, use needles to drain fluids from a chest, and administer a wide range of medications.

Structured medical evacuation with trained nurses is a new phenomenon, dating back to only 1985. For about fifteen years before that, nurses would accompany patients on commercial or transport flights, but the service was haphazard. Prior to that, there were dogsleds, and long waits for flights. A trip from Whale Cove to Rankin Inlet, only seventy-six kilometres as the goose flies, could take fourteen days; now it takes minutes by plane.

The single most common reason for transporting a person out of a northern community is respiratory problems. Next are obstetrical cases, followed by those afflicted with heart disease and victims of various sorts of trauma. It is important for a nurse to know the societal factors involved in these cases. For a variety of reasons—poorly ventilated homes, smoking rates, use of oil lamps, a highly sociable culture—RSV* flourishes in the North. Every

---

* RSV, or respiratory syncytial virus, is the name given a group of myxoviruses responsible for infections such as bronchopneumonia, bronchiolitis, and the common cold. It is particularly dangerous to children.

couple of years, there is an epidemic that claims several children's lives; in 1997, for example, Keewatin evacuated 109 children in just four weeks. Among the elderly, there is a high incidence of congenital heart defects that lead to chronic heart and lung problems, which are exacerbated by social and environmental conditions. And the combination of frightening rates of sexually transmitted diseases (STDs) and smoking helps explain the obstetrics cases; STDs can lead to ectopic pregnancies (in which the fertilized egg implants outside the uterus), and smoking to low birth weight and premature babies. While guns are plentiful, shooting accidents are almost unheard of; there is a building boom in Nunavut and most traumas are related to construction, or to house fires.

More than half the patients evacuated from the territory annually are children, and one in five is a birthing mother, so flight nurses need a good grounding in pediatrics and obstetrics. They also need nerves of steel—northern flights in the winter are never smooth— and ample flexibility. Emergency care is never easy, but it is doubly difficult in a plane during turbulence, or in the back of a pickup truck in the dead of winter. In fact, one of the major headaches of medical evacuation is getting the patients from the nursing station (or wherever else they may be in distress) to the airplane. In all of Nunavut, there is one ambulance, and it is in Rankin Inlet. Everywhere else, the nurses borrow pickup trucks or snowmobiles.

The weather is always a factor. An intravenous line can freeze up, a trachial tube can snap off, and incubator batteries last only minutes in the bitter cold. In these conditions, nurses get creative. Drugs are always administered by infusion pump, and an incubator coat is fashioned out of Thinsulate and Velcro. The policy is to stabilize patients as much as possible before moving them. When they head to the airport, the plane is running, and the transfer is immediate. "What we always do is minimize the time outside," Triggs says. This is true for the planes too; in the extreme cold, an aircraft that spends too much time on the ground may not be able to take off again, so pilots get in and out quickly.

The reality, however, is that there are many days in the North when flying is impossible. Winter lasts from October until June, and storms shut down airports for several days each month. Even during the summer, communities on the shores of Hudson Bay can become fog-bound. "The tragedies that we do have are all due to weather, stuff like an ectopic pregnancy or a woman with heavy antepartum bleeding that you just can't move because of a storm. In those situations, you're just powerless," Triggs says.

Once the plane is in the air, there are many complications as well, even on a smooth ride. The planes are specially modified for medical transport, but routine nursing tasks are still difficult because of lack of space; gas expands at high altitudes, so adjustments have to be made to oxygen; and nurses get only one chance to pack all the supplies they might need. Some patients have never been in a plane, and their reactions are unpredictable.

Triggs stresses that team work is essential, that flight nurses could not do their jobs without the superb pilots that ferry them around. For example, when oxygen is needed, nurses will ask for an altitude restriction, meaning that the flight stays low. And she says nurses still do not get enough recognition for specialized skills they need to do the job. When she began lobbying to have flight nursing recognized as a distinct nursing specialty in 1987, Triggs says, she was told it was nothing more than a "hand-holding, babysitting service" that required no special talent. She set out to change that view, travelling all over Canada and the United States to study air-ambulance services. Her research, from which she concluded that medical evacuation in the North was well intentioned but poorly planned and delivered, helped change the business dramatically. Now, not only are the services better administered, but every nurse gets specialized training.

When Triggs trains flight nurses, she stresses preparation and planning, that the ideal evacuation is one in which the nurse does virtually nothing in the air. "Let's face it; the airplane is not a good place to be delivering premature babies or to be defribilating," she points out. In fact, Triggs gets angry at stories that romanticize nurses and doctors who do complex life-saving manoeuvres aboard air ambulances. "When I hear about a company that had four deliveries and a cardiac arrest in one week, I see that as bad planning. I wouldn't want to be on one of their flights. We don't want heroics, we want good nursing care."

Yet, even with the best-laid plans, the occasional emergency does occur. In Nunavut and Manitoba,* government policy is to have only one nurse aboard a medical-evacuation flight (though, in rare cases, they may have a physician along). Triggs finds this approach, designed to save money, troubling because "in an emergency, one pair of hands is not enough."

When she left the Manitoba Air Ambulance service for Keewatin Air in 1993, Triggs was, as a nurse, ambivalent about working for a for-profit company in the health-care sector, but her view has changed since then. "We don't ever compromise to save money, because our reputation depends on quality. That can't be said about the public health-care system anymore. They compromise; they cut corners all the time, to save money," she complains.

While Keewatin Air's government contracts are significant—it works in Nunavut, Manitoba, and Saskatchewan—most of its medical evacuations are carried out for insurance companies. It also has a division called Critical Care International that does medical transport to Europe, Asia, and Africa. In fact, the morning of a scheduled interview, Triggs was awoken at 5:00 A.M. by a client who wanted to get a patient from Arizona to Switzerland.† The plane's crew, including two nurses, was ready to go at 8:00 A.M. "That's really the big challenge in this job. There's a lot of organizational details to get done in three hours to prepare for a twenty-five-hour mission," she says.

* Every province and territory (except Newfoundland and Prince Edward Island) has a medical-evacuation service (a combination of government agencies and contracts with private companies).
† Keewatin's business is booming because, if you look at global air routes, you will see that Winnipeg is an ideal base from which to make such flights quickly and cheaply. Most governments and private insurers try to repatriate sick patients from abroad quickly because of the exorbitant costs charged in the United States.

Yet, the skills that Triggs acquired long ago in the intensive-care unit and refined over the years—thinking on her feet, remaining calm, constantly reassessing and planning—are those that have helped her succeed not only as a flight nurse, but as a business person. Many nurses who are bored and frustrated could find an important lesson in Triggs's story. "This started out as an adventure, something new. But flight nursing has opened a whole new world to me, one that is full of opportunities. I do stuff now that I could never have dreamed of doing in a hospital."

It Looks Like Child's Play— Claire Sheinman Cowan

Dealing with the non-life-threatening aches and pains of children— the tonsillectomies, hernias, broken bones, and infections that are part of growing up—is often seen as one of the easiest jobs in the nursing world.

"Well, have you ever tried to take the vital signs of a three-year-old who has decided he doesn't want to play that game?" asks Claire Sheinman Cowan, with a knowing chuckle. "Whatever time you think it should take for a procedure, quadruple it for children, because they can be creative in their resistance."

The reality, Cowan says, is not that pediatrics is easy, but that good nurses make the job look easy. The really important work nurses do is low-tech; it's subtle and hidden. Pediatric nursing is about noticing little changes in a condition, intervening creatively, and supporting families in a time of need.

Good pediatric nurses are able to laugh and play at the same time as they perform deadly serious work, such as assessing symptoms and giving injections. They are also unpretentious and relate easily to children. "If you're intimidated by the idea of doing your job while wearing a Snuggly, or if you don't like dressing up and making funny voices, you're probably not a good fit here," Cowan says.

As program-development manager for the pediatrics department at St. Joseph's Health Centre in Toronto, Cowan faced the challenge of building a department almost from scratch. In this era of cutbacks and retrenchment, she is swimming against the current, dramatically expanding a program. Assigning such an administrative task to a nurse is a relatively new phenomenon, but a trend that is catching on. More and more often, hospitals are turning to nurses for administrative functions, in particular, program development, because nurses have sound clinical knowledge, administrative abilities, and a rapport with the health-care consumer.

Nursing, which demands well-honed decision-making and analytical skills, also attracts those with natural leadership skills. Good nurses are also skilled communicators, a must at a time when consumers are demanding more input into health care and when institutions are reaching out to the community for support, financial and otherwise.

Cowan says there are many advantages to being a nurse, even in a largely administrative position. "Some things that I do, you don't have to be a nurse. But the core of my work—establishing practice standards, equipment standards, and hiring—would be impossible without my nursing background. Let me put it another way: when there was leadership provided by people who were not pediatric nurses, you could really see the gaps." As an added bonus, St. Joseph's gets a manager who can pitch in at bedside when it gets busy. "I'm on call seven days a week, twenty-four hours a day. As a manager, I feel I have to make that commitment to my staff. And I get called a lot, especially in the peak winter season," Cowan notes.

Under Ontario's hospitals restructuring program—which, despite much opposition and some excesses, brought in some positive and long-overdue administrative reforms and creative new jobs—St. Joseph's became a regional pediatrics centre for western Toronto, a full-fledged centre that is no longer the perennial poor cousin to the Hospital for Sick Children (often called "Sick Kids"). What was created, instead, was the Child Health Network, with

Sick Kids as the hub and beefed-up regional programs throughout the Greater Toronto Area.

Cowan's job is to take a moribund, second-class pediatrics unit with fourteen beds and transform it into a regional centre with thirty-eight beds, an emergency department, an active day-surgery program, and an ambitious family-life health centre. That means upgrading everything—staff, equipment, and facilities. It also means learning to serve a local community, a skill that hospitals have forgotten in recent years. St. Joseph's straddles High Park, a middle-class neighbourhood, and Parkdale, a working-class area, both of them home to a culturally diverse population.

Cowan, an American who came to Canada almost two decades ago, uses a hockey metaphor to explain her approach to such a daunting task: "It's the Wayne Gretzky school of nursing. I'm never looking to see where the puck is, I'm heading to where the puck is going. If you want to offer the best programs, you have to remain that one step ahead. . . . For once, I get to, not call all the shots, but . . . build a new program based on nursing standards."

One of her most difficult tasks is hiring. Shortages mean that nurses, particularly those in specialized fields, can pick and choose. In pediatrics, the summit is Sick Kids, so St. Joseph's is always competing at a slight disadvantage. Sick Kids also has distinct practical advantages; as a unionized workplace, St. Joseph's is bound by collective agreements, which, among other things, make it impossible to offer signing bonuses. Sick Kids, whose nurses do not belong to the Ontario Nurses Association, routinely offers enticing cash payments when it has a position to fill.

"The pitch I make is that, in our program, you can chart your own course, while, at Sick Kids, you're just one of many. This is the farm club for managers-to-be, it's a place where you can get the experience to move to the next level," Cowan points out.

What qualities does she look for? A pediatric nurse must have not only patience, but a personality that kids are comfortable with, Cowan says, as well as other necessary traits that would be considered unusual in many workplaces, such as "being a goofball."

On a more serious note, Cowan is blunt about an issue that most managers will discuss only in hushed tones. "In community hospitals, nurses are too old. I'm the average age of a bedside nurse [45], and that's too old. We need new blood." This is particularly true in pediatrics, a specialty where nurses tend to stay until retirement, and where you need a lot of energy to keep up with the patients.

The problem, according to Cowan, is that nursing has never received its due. Like every other female-dominated profession, it is undervalued and underpaid. "Society does not value what we do. It does not value caring; it values things like science and technology," Cowan says.

"The true value of the time that a nurse spends with a child and his family is not easily quantifiable. You write in the log: 'One hour of providing support.' But those words are so inadequate. They in no way capture what a nurse has done. She may have dramatically changed the health outcome; she may have saved a life. But no one ever measures that, no one ever puts it into words."

A Healthy Start—Paula Robeson

"It often astounds me that I can have an impact, that I can contribute in some small way to a change that will benefit children forever," says Paula Robeson. As director of early childhood development at the Canadian Institute of Child Health, she is fashioning the policy changes of tomorrow that will have long-lasting repercussions and help provide all Canadian children with the best future possible.

Every time you see an infant buckled into a car seat, a toddler wearing flame-resistant pyjamas, or a child strapping on a bicycle helmet, you are witnessing a nurse's work. Health-promotion nurses have contributed to the dramatic decrease in the incidence of low-birth-weight babies, developed sexual-abuse-prevention programs, helped change the way parents discipline their children, and been on the front lines of the vaccination revolution.

These changes in legislation and in public attitudes did not come about magically, but through the tireless work of advocates like those at the institute, who, during the past two decades, have quietly led the charge on most of these issues. But much of their work goes unrecognized.

"Where we see a service gap, a knowledge gap, or a policy gap, we try to figure out how that gap can best be closed," says Robeson, a former neonatal nurse. That means being acutely aware of trends and issues as they arise in the media, in peer-reviewed journals, on the Internet, and in neighbourhoods.

Robeson focuses primarily on the 0-to-6 age group, among whom the leading cause of death is falls, usually in ordinary household accidents, and among whom there is still a high number of preventable disabilities. Two of the greatest dangers to the fetus, for example, are alcohol and cigarette smoke. Robeson actively develops programs to get pregnant moms to quit smoking (and also not to resume after the birth, because more than 200 children a year in Canada die from illnesses linked to exposure to second-hand smoke) and to prevent and treat fetal alcohol syndrome. She is also working on an awareness program about the importance of folic acid for pregnant women; ensuring an adequate supply of the nutrient in an expectant mother's diet can virtually eliminate the risk of spina bifida (a congenital defect affecting the development of one or more vertebrae).

Over the years, the institute has made its name with its injury-prevention initiatives. Seat belts, infant car seats, and bike helmets, whose use is now second nature for most children, were unheard of a generation ago. Pyjamas were made of highly flammable material until the institute lobbied for regulatory changes after the horrific deaths of a number of children. After news of choking deaths, it pushed for better regulation and labelling of toys. Much of that role now rests with Safe Kids Canada, a charitable group that focuses strictly on injury-prevention initiatives. Today, the Institute of Child Health directs more of its efforts towards environmental-health issues, such as the effects of low-level chemical exposure on child development, and a broad range of parenting issues.

"Our definition of health includes not only physical health, but well-being and mental health. And I don't mean mental illness; I mean kids' happiness, self-esteem, social interaction, their environment, and their community. Growing into independent young men and women in Canada today requires us to pay attention to the whole gamut," Robeson explains.

The institute has a multidisciplinary team (featuring three nurses) that spends a lot of time brainstorming and exchanging ideas. Out of these informal talks come more detailed program ideas. Robeson will do research, build alliances with groups with similar interests, and write proposals for funding. She also does a lot of public advocacy and lobbying, with groups ranging from parent associations to Senate committees. All this, naturally, entails a lot of meetings and correspondence, much of it with government policy-makers.

"When I went to nursing school, I never dreamed of doing this kind of work—of spending a lot of time at a desk, writing reports. But the career choices I made along the way have brought me to this point," Robeson says. While she occasionally misses the hands-on aspect of nursing in an institutional or community setting, she feels the backroom work she does is invaluable, and rewarding: "When you get through and a policy changes, that feels really good."

It is her experience in the trenches, from a neonatal intensive-care unit in St. John's to a community-health clinic for children in Vancouver, that has made her appreciate and understand policy formulation. She realizes that the overall health of Canadian children requires front-line nurses in hospitals and the community, health-promotion nurses, policy-makers, advocates. While her specialty is young children, much of her role as an advocate is more fundamental, promoting the value of health promotion itself. "Nursing is a very economical way of doing health promotion. If you prevent one case of fetal alcohol syndrome, if you stop one new mother from smoking, or you prevent a major disability because a kid is wearing a bike helmet, the savings for that one child are going to be enormous, plus there are going to be positive repercussions, on the entire household and even parts of the community," she says. Unfortunately, the public and politicians are a lot more excited by the technology in a hospital than by health-promotion campaigns that keep kids out of hospital.

Nevertheless, the job is a satisfying one, Robeson adds, because she sees the organization's policies affecting her own children every day. For example, her daughter's school has come on board the "safe routes to school" project, a campaign to minimize the risks children face walking to school. While most parents cite "stranger danger" (the fear of a sexual predator) as their primary concern, the real risk to their children's well-being comes from drivers who speed and ignore stop signs. The institute believes most parents overestimate the ability of their children to deal with those risks and advocates environmental changes (traffic calming, law enforcement, walking school buses)* to reduce risks. It is a tough sell in a world that values speediness.

Increasingly, the Institute of Child Health is embracing theories such as "determinants of health," the belief that factors such as income, diet, social status, and birth weight can predict future health outcomes. These matters come naturally to nurses, who have always had a holistic view of health. At the institute, the role of nurses such as Robeson is to make these complex notions understandable. " 'Determinants of health' is not a term that is understood by most people, so you have to make the jargon family-friendly. Anyone can understand that if Johnny eats breakfast, he will be happier and more attentive in school, and that means he's more likely to stay in school longer, and ultimately that means he's more likely to get a good job," she says. But each of those steps implies a need for supportive policies.

Changing the workplace to make it more family-friendly is one of the institute's major policy initiatives of the future, and it

* In some urban neighbourhoods, parents are banding together so their children can walk to school together, in a supervised fashion, a tactic dubbed the "walking school bus."

preaches by example. Despite being a small organization, it allows job sharing and flexible work hours, is accommodating when children are sick, welcomes them in the office, allows employees to be available to their children during the so-called witching hour (the 3:00-to-5:00 P.M. period between the end of the school day and the end of most workdays), and has a buddy system so that someone knowledgeable and supportive can always take a call even if a parent is absent from the office. In fact, as a health-promotion nurse, Robeson works three days a week—by choice—with no shift work, no weekends, and no beeper. It is the antithesis to most nurses' working conditions.

"I've worked in a lot of places that practised medicine, but where employees were unhealthy. Here, they promote health in every sense of the word, and that's stimulating," she says. But one thing Robeson shares with many other nurses is the precariousness of her work. "This is a non-profit group with no core funding. If the grants don't come, there will be no jobs. I think the days are gone when a nurse can say her job is forever."

Part Two
CHILDHOOD
TO ADOLESCENCE

A Shining Morning Face

In stark contrast to early childhood, the school years are the healthiest of our lives. The 5-to-14 age group distinguishes itself with the lowest death rate and lowest hospitalization rate. But, at the same time, it is a time of dramatic emotional development, when children learn to become independent

The school years are a time of learning, not only in the classroom, but socially. It is also a time when young people develop habits, good and bad, that will affect their health for a lifetime—and, by extension, the health-care system.

Joan Mikkelsen is a school nurse. Her eloquent description of primary school today, of the health challenges that children face daily—the pressure to smoke, to drink, to have sex, is ever-present from Grade 4 on—should convince policy-makers that school nursing is one of the best investments we can make as a society.

The school nurse has promoted hygiene since "Red Cross hour" was instituted in the classroom during the Second World War. Today, school nurses like Mikkelsen play an important role in preventing the spread of infectious disease (through vaccination programs), in preventing child abuse, and in trying to control what has become the scourge of childhood—respiratory diseases such as asthma. A whopping 13 per cent of boys and 11 per cent of girls—more than 90,000 Canadian children in total—are believed to suffer from asthma. The disease also accounts for more than half of all hospitalizations among children.

Yet, sadly, while they are needed more than ever, school nurses are a dying breed. Where the positions exist, nurses are responsible for about a dozen schools each, in addition to other duties in the community. Education systems do not want to pay for any health costs, and public health tends to be a municipal responsibility. With provinces dumping costs on municipalities, one of the first cuts made is public health, and, because children do not have a voice, they suffer.

We have allowed ourselves to be blinded by our children's outward appearance of physical health. Most children—save the 10 per cent or so with physical disabilities—run and play, laugh and sing. They appear carefree. Yet one in every five children has a diagnosable mental-health problem. One of the leading causes of death among children 10 and older is suicide. In fact, it is second only to motor-vehicle accidents.

Cars and trucks with reckless drivers at the wheel account for two of every three deaths and injuries among school-age children. The tragic reality is that, while many parents worry about perverts and child molesters in their neighbourhoods, the greatest risk to their children is the driver who is pressured or distracted and speeds or runs a stop sign.

It is easy to blame children—and police tend to, particularly when investigating the cases of pedestrians who are struck down—but most simply do not have the motor skills to deal with traffic that moves at the pace it does today. What is required to make our communities safe for children is environmental change such as traffic-calming measures and, above all, enforcement of existing traffic rules by police.

Children in Canada are four times more likely to die in traffic accidents—virtually all of them preventable—than they are to die of childhood cancers. Yet we can not ignore the devastation wrought by cancer.

You will meet pediatric-oncology nurse Kim Widger. Her work

is bittersweet. There are few things sadder than a child who is suffering a painful death. At the same time, advances in this field have been so spectacular that most children now survive cancer, which was once an automatic death sentence. Oncology nurses have to provide a combination of pure caregiving—the hand-holding and hugging that are often more valuable than any medicine—and technical knowledge that has to be continually updated.

This is a mixed blessing. Many pediatric cancer patients are now joining the ranks of the chronically ill. There are thousands of children with chronic illnesses, both physical and mental, such as Down syndrome, spina bifida, hemophilia, muscular dystrophy, and diabetes. Most of them get regular nursing care. There are children today who require around-the-clock care, such as the ventilator-dependent, who used to be confined to institutions but now can remain home, thanks to nursing. This is an important but neglected area of nursing care.

In Part Two, we also meet cystic-fibrosis-clinic nurse Anne Gold. She deals with a particularly difficult clientele who have been relatively healthy throughout childhood but often have to face their mortality when they reach adolescence. She provides not only medical care, but guidance on how to cope with socially devastating disabilities.

The care Gold provides—hands-on, holistic, and heartfelt—is a model for the way we should all be, and expect to be, treated. For her, treating the disease is secondary; what matters most is promoting, and revelling in, wellness.

Gold works at the renowned Hospital for Sick Children in Toronto. When Sick Kids opened on March 23, 1875, it had one nurse, one matron, and one servant (no doctors!). The first patient was a girl who had been scalded by boiling water. Today, it is one of the most modern pediatric facilities in the world, but nurses are still the backbone, as they are in most health-care institutions.

During the school years, one in every twenty children will be hospitalized, with the leading causes being tonsillectomy and asthma treatment. There are more than 535,000 children and teenagers with disabilities in Canada, about 7 per cent of that population. Three-quarters of these young people have chronic, long-term conditions that challenge not only the health-care system, but our notions of integration and belonging in society.

As our health-care system becomes more consumer-oriented (again, thanks in large part to nurses), people will increasingly be demanding sound, accessible health information for their families. Telehealth nurse Catherine Bowness is on the front lines in the struggle to meet that demand. She takes calls, many of them from parents, looking for advice on all kinds of everyday health concerns.

Nurses have long been there to treat the aches and pains of childhood. Today, they do so with increasing specialization, but without losing sight of the basics, the holistic approach to caring that is key to transforming the illness-care system into a true health-care system.

A Dying Breed—Joan Mikkelsen

With 518 children, Ocean View Elementary School in Eastern Passage, Nova Scotia, is bustling and bursting at the seams. Kids in this age group, 5 to 10, tend to be daring and rambunctious, so there is a steady stream of cuts, bruises, and broken bones. "We go through more ice than a downtown bar," jokes the principal, Brenda Waterman.

But children suffer from a lot more than scraped knees and black eyes. A sign on the front door warns that the school is "scent-free," meaning visitors wearing perfume or cologne or having washed with scented soap are unwelcome. Peanuts in any form, including the old staple, peanut butter and jelly sandwiches, are strictly banned. Twenty-five per cent of students have asthma and need puffers. As many again take Ritalin. An even larger number have allergies, more than a handful of them of the life-threatening variety. A few have diabetes; a couple more, epilepsy. Two have Tourette's syndrome. One girl has a serious heart condition.

Another is partially paralysed. Until recently, there was a severely handicapped boy in a wheelchair, but he moved. In other words, it is a fairly typical Canadian school.

And, like most schools today, Ocean View does not have a full-time school nurse. Management of this litany of medical conditions falls on teachers and the principal, who are overwhelmed by it all. To underscore the point, Waterman lifts a large Rubbermaid box onto her desk and peels off the lid. It is full of puffers, epi-pens,* and medications, each item identified with a child's name and all of them cross-referenced on an accompanying sheet. Then she points to a series of photos on the wall of high-risk kids, featuring detailed descriptions of their conditions—peanut allergy, allergy to new-car smell, grand mal seizures, and so on—and appropriate emergency interventions.

"All I can say is: 'Thank God we can call Joan for help,'" Waterman sighs. Joan Mikkelsen is a public-health nurse with the Central Regional Health Board in Nova Scotia. She is responsible for nine schools (seven elementary and two junior high) located around the eastern shore of Halifax Harbour, and a clinic at a local parent resource centre. With thousands of students under her care, she cannot possibly attend to every injury, case of anaphylactic shock, or infectious disease. She concentrates instead on prevention, and on teaching the basics of better health. "We would love to be in every school every day, there's so much work to do. It would pay off very quickly in public-health savings, but hiring public-health nurses is, unfortunately, not a political priority," Mikkelsen points out.

The core of her work is immunization and vision care. In Nova Scotia, all students have their eyes tested when they begin kindergarten. Nurses are looking principally for a condition called "lazy eye," which can lead to blindness. All Grade 4 students are also vaccinated against hepatitis B, a disease transmitted through bodily

* Epinephrine, a powerful hormone, is sometimes used to dilate bronchial airways. A device called an epi-pen is often used to inject the drug to counteract allergic reactions.

fluids that can cause severe liver problems, and 15-year-olds get a booster to protect them against tetanus, a bacteria that can destroy the central nervous system. Aside from that, Mikkelsen has great leeway to respond to the needs of students and teachers as she sees fit, and her work ranges from teaching parenting skills through to consulting about the architectural designs of schools.

In elementary school, the nurse teaches about hygiene, particularly hand-washing. Mikkelsen will bring in an ultraviolet light to show kids the germs on their hands, a gimmick they love. Ocean View, a modern school, has a sink in every classroom, a public-health innovation nurses pushed for. Dirty hands are the principal means of transmitting respiratory diseases such as the flu and the common cold, and U.S. studies have shown that regular hand-washing dramatically cuts absenteeism among students and staff.

Mikkelsen also teaches about safety and promotes the wearing of bicycle helmets. To drive home the point, she fills a balloon with grape Jell-O so that it weighs about 1 kilogram, the same weight and consistency as the brain, and drops it to the floor: the splatter says it all. One of her pet projects is lobbying the local school board to replace schoolyard asphalt with grass, a move she feels would dramatically reduce injuries such as concussions and broken bones.

With older children, the emphasis is on sexuality, growth and development, and nutrition. One of the most troubling trends she has seen is a significant rise in eating disorders among young girls. Mikkelsen feels no-nonsense education about sex is a public-health necessity because, by grades 5 and 6, many students are already experimenting with smoking, drinking, and sexual activity, and pretending otherwise will not change that fact. "Teachers use us as a buffer, for introducing notions that they know should be raised but might upset parents," Mikkelsen says.

At junior high schools, the nurse is also called upon to teach about health and sexuality, but the lessons are more explicit. Mikkelsen tackles birth control, sexually transmitted diseases, date rape, building healthy relationships, and social issues such as drug and alcohol use. She also does a lot of counselling, because students feel more comfortable talking to a nurse than to a teacher.

Mikkelsen is constantly firefighting. She gets about 100 calls a week from teachers and principals during the school year on every health issue imaginable: a kindergarten child who wets his pants; a kid with scabies; a child who faints in class because she is not fed breakfast; a child who needs tube feeding; an outbreak of measles; a bully who steals other kids' asthma puffers; a young boy who is sexually aggressive; a bright student whose marks have plummeted because her parents split up.

In many cases, the nurse will make house calls to discuss sensitive issues with parents. "A visit from a nurse is a lot less threatening than one from a social worker," Mikkelsen says. In most cases, there is no malice on the part of the parents, they are just overwhelmed. "Parenting is an area that needs a lot more attention than it gets. When parents have questions, they really have nowhere to turn," she says.

What do parents call her about most? "Head lice generates, by far, the most calls, but it's nothing but a nuisance," Mikkelsen says. (Three times a year, parent-volunteers do screening in elementary schools to keep them nit-free.) "It's too bad parents don't have a better sense of the public-health issues that really affect their children. Motor-vehicle accidents are the number one killer of chidren, but parents get more worked up about lice than about speeding."

Surprisingly, many teachers also call with personal health concerns. The average age of teachers in Canada is 45—the same as for nurses—and they have questions about menopause, breast cancer, infertility, and coping with stress.

Mikkelsen realizes that in many parts of the country the school nurse is a dying breed, but hopes that health administrators and educators will come to their senses and realize the great return on investment from early intervention. "These kids are a captive audience and they're eager to learn. The habits they develop in elementary school stay with them for life," she notes. Mikkelsen has fond memories of the school nurse in her home town of East Glace Bay. "I can remember her quite clearly. Mrs. Guthrie was her name. I even remember the way she wore her hair." She laughs. But, more important was the role the nurse played in community development—after all, everybody in town knew the nurse—instilling healthy habits early, and inspiring young girls like Joan Mikkelsen to embark on a career in public-health nursing.

How Do You Answer "Why?"?—Kim Widger

"Your child has cancer."

It is a statement that every parent dreads. But Kim Widger has heard it hundreds of times in her work as a pediatric-oncology nurse at Alberta Children's Hospital in Calgary.*

"Often the parents are in such shock that they don't hear anything after 'Your child has cancer.' That's why nurses are in the meeting where the diagnosis is given, because we have to answer all the questions that come up later."

While oncologists deliver the bad news, and determine the protocols for treating cancer, it is nurses who administer most of the hands-on physical and emotional care for the sick child and the family. It is gruelling, emotional work, but strangely uplifting.

According to the Canadian Cancer Society, almost 900 Canadian children annually find out that they have cancer, and the disease accounts for about one in five pediatric deaths, or about 175 children, each year. Medical advances, particularly in early diagnosis techniques, mean that the survival rate is now close to 75 per cent for kids with cancer. Those with Hodgkin's disease (a malignancy of the lymph glands) or a Wilm's tumour (on the kidney) now have a 90 per cent survival rate; at the other end of the scale are brain tumours, the majority of which are still fatal.

Widger says each form of cancer—and she can rhyme off almost fifty in rapid-fire fashion—poses particular challenges for a nurse.

* Widger has since moved to Halifax to start a pediatric palliative-care program at Izaak Walton Killam–Grace Health Centre.

Children with brain tumours often suffer dramatic personality changes and can be violent; those who undergo amputation or disfiguring surgery can be extremely depressed; and those who receive bone-marrow transplants become violently ill. Similarly, parents go through a full range of emotions, particularly when the prognosis is grim.

"We're the ones who are there at 3:00 A.M. when Mom can't sleep and she has a million questions. Three or four in the morning is when you have the deep conversations about the meaning of life," Widger says.

Alberta Children's Hospital has eleven beds in its oncology unit, but it has had up to double that number of children in active treatment at one time. Generally, the nurse to patient ratio is two to one, though one to one care is the norm for palliative-care and bone-marrow-transplant patients. The bulk of work done by oncology nurses revolves around the administration of drugs and ongoing asssessment that takes place during these tasks.

"Chemotherapy" is a catch-all term for the treatment of disease by chemical agents. They can be administered in a number of ways: injection (either push or intravenous drip) into a central line or into the spine, or even orally. On Widger's unit, there are fifteen to twenty chemotherapy treatments* used routinely, in addition to radiotherapy and a bevy of supportive drugs such as painkillers, antibiotics, antifungals, anti-rejection drugs, steroids, nutritional supplements, stool softeners, and blood products.

Nurses not only have to be familiar with all these drugs, but also must understand their side effects and the combinations used in various treatment protocols. And they always have to be aware of up-to-the-minute information because the parents keep them on their toes; "they get on the Internet and then ask incredibly detailed questions," Widger says.

In fact, one of Widger's principal roles is education of the parents

* Anti-cancer drugs generally inhibit the proliferation of cells. They include alkylating agents, antimetabolites, periwinkle plant derivatives, antineoplastic antibiotics, and radioactive isotopes.

and children. They need to be taught to care for a central line, a plastic tube that is inserted in the chest, arm, or neck to allow easy administration of drugs. They need to learn about the risks of infection during chemotherapy, and the importance of good nutrition for a child with cancer. And because some treatments, such as those for leukemia, can last up to three years, many parents want to know minute details of treatment protocols.

The magical moments, Widger says, rarely come during the hustle and bustle of daily treatment: instead, they occur when the child has some quiet time alone with the nurse. The children will take the intimate moments to ask a nurse to buy one last present for their mother before they die or to ask some difficult questions.

"They always want to know how it is to die, how it feels. They also want to know why they got cancer. How do you answer 'Why?'? 'Honestly,' I say, 'I don't know.' I tell them: 'I wish I could take the cancer away from you, but I can't.' Kids know there is no answer to that question, so I don't try to make one up. But what I do stress is that it's not their fault. You have to tell them, specially the young ones, that it's not because they hit their brother or called their mom a bad name. It's just because," she says.

Widger has had more than two decades of experience in pediatric oncology, but she is the exception. There is a disproportionate number of young nurses in the field because of the emotional demands. Many nurses cannot face the job after they have children themselves. And the majority work in the area part-time, again because it is too hard to work with suffering and dying children day after day.

Widger says the most difficult part of the job for her is not the palliative cases, but those where the treatment is devastating, such as a bone-marrow transplant. Before the transplant itself—which is actually an injection—there is a week-long preparation that consists of three days of radiation and three days of very intense chemotherapy (three or four times the regular-strength dose). Many children start vomiting at the door, and do not stop for weeks; their body is wracked with pain as the drugs essentially destroy the immune system to prevent the body from rejecting the donor marrow. For many kids, the worst part is the mouth sores that develop; their mouths tend to look like raw hamburger. Then, to top it all off, the marrow itself smells disgusting (like rotting oysters). "As a nurse, you feel powerless," Widger says quietly.

Yet, the palliative cases, where all treatments have failed and cancer is going to kill the child, the nurse finds easier because she feels more able to make a tangible difference as a caregiver. "I know that this will sound strange to anyone who's not a palliative nurse, but watching kids die is not depressing, it's a very special experience. As a nurse, my role is not to do the impossible, to create a miracle, it's to make it a good death," Widger says.

The media portrayal of children with terminal cancer is that of heroic figures who are at peace with themselves. Widger agrees. In her experience, children never really give up, but they also tend to realize when their time is at an end. For her, one of the most remarkable parts of the job is seeing a child plan his own funeral, give away all his belongings, comfort his parents, then go home to die.

Experiencing that intimacy is the reason Widger says she has never wished to be a physician rather than a nurse. "I've spent seven years in university. I could be a doctor. But I choose not to be. If I was a physician, I couldn't walk in to the room of a kid who's awake at three in the morning and say: 'Hi, how are you?' I could never be at the bedside when they take their last breath. That's the privilege of being a nurse. I know these kids, I care for these kids, in a way a physician could never dream of doing. When you realize that, why would you want to be anything but a nurse?"

Lives in a Hurry—Anne Gold

For many, the image of cystic fibrosis (CF) is of a sallow-faced child sitting down with a bowl full of pills while a solemn-sounding voiceover declares that this is the medication required for the child to be able to eat a meal. That haunting television fundraising plea fades in the waiting room of the CF Clinic at Toronto's Hospital for

Sick Children. You would never know that the gurgling babies, children colouring in books, and fidgeting teenagers are all afflicted with a chronic, always fatal, lung disease.*

Anne Gold, a clinical nurse-specialist and nurse-practitioner at the clinic, speaks proudly of the track-and-field champs, Ontario scholars, and Kiwanis Festival winners who are her patients, and of their dreams, aspirations, growing independence, and budding sexuality.

"I focus on what's happening in their lives, not their lungs, but the two are intertwined. These kids have a lot of living to do, and they're in a hurry," she says. Though Gold sees CF patients ranging from newborns to 18-year-olds, her love is adolescents.

They can be obnoxious, brooding, insecure, and awkward. For a public-health nurse, they can be a nightmare because they generally hate to listen and love to take risks. But when you get through, when you make the connection, they are so full of passion and energy that it makes it all worthwhile, Gold says. "Either you love working with adolescents or you hate it. Those of us with a rebellious side enjoy the challenge."

Doubly challenging is the fact that these teenagers have been surrounded by the medical system their entire lives. They are tired of being poked and prodded, and resent being treated as "sick kids" instead of as grown-ups. Conscious of this, Gold began her job at the clinic by asking for new furniture. The pediatric table and chairs that are standard issue at Sick Kids were replaced with full-size models in a couple of rooms. And once the patients hit 12 or 13 years of age, she asks parents to remain in the waiting room during visits.

"Because they have been coming here so long, it's easy to forget they are budding adults. I focus on them becoming more independent, on making their own decisions. I like to see them alone, so they can speak more freely—much to the chagrin of their parents," she says with a chuckle.

---

* CF is an inherited disease (both parents must carry the gene) that is usually diagnosed in childhood. A simple sweat test is used, as sufferers have high levels of sodium and chloride in their perspiration.

CF kids visit the clinic every three months for routine check-ups, and once a year they will get a full work-over. Many will also spend time in hospital getting treatment for lung infections. Gold does a physical exam, one that is directed towards cystic fibrosis. She teaches about medication and physiotherapy, both of which are regular fixtures in her patients' lives. As a nurse-practitioner, she can do some limited prescribing, and order tests without getting the approval of a physician. Doctors also refer patients to her because they are not as adept at dealing with the psychosocial aspects of the disease. That is where Gold places her emphasis during clinic visits, which last at least an hour.

"I start every visit by saying: 'Tell me about your life since we last met.' I tend to be quite social with my kids. Schmoozing is a big part of what I do," she says. Gold will also meet them outside the hospital, on their own turf—at home or at the mall. They will talk about school, sports, new boyfriends or girlfriends, but almost never about the disease.

"The most important thing I do is not listening to their lungs, it's listening to what they have to say. Nobody ever asks adolescents what they care about. The most important question I ask of this age group is: 'What do you do for fun?'" Gold says. A response like "I don't have any friends" or "I'm too tired to do anything" can reveal health problems more serious than the patient lets on, or shame about the disease.

CF is a debilitating disease. The glands of young sufferers become clogged with thick mucus, especially in the lungs, pancreas, and intestines. The pills they take before meals are enzymes to help them digest fat. They also take significant amounts of antibiotics to fight off respiratory infections, which are common and ultimately fatal. Because of the stress on the pancreas, many CF patients also develop diabetes. The dream of many is a double lung transplant, but the waiting lists are long. "In the clinic, each time you hear a trauma coded, you say: 'Maybe that's Joseph's lungs.'" While Gold has become a big promoter of organ donation, she recognizes the best hope is a cure. To that end, she does some volunteer work with the Canadian Cystic Fibrosis Foundation, which supports research, and participates in its fundraising events, such as the Zellers Moonwalk. (It is interesting that, under the influence of people with chronic diseases and those who work closely with them such as nurses, the old fundraising images of sufferers as pathetic and hopeless have been replaced by much more positive ones.)

While the old TV spot is no longer accurate—drugs are more powerful and compact now—medication is still an issue with many self-conscious teens. Popping three pills before downing a slice of pizza with friends can provoke so many questions that they will simply skip the essential treatment. Gold wrote her master's thesis on body image among adolescents with chronic disease, and that knowledge serves her well. Because of fat-absorption problems, kids with CF are rail-thin and that, ironically, "gives girls bodies that many of their peers would kill for. I really have to watch them because they will skip the medication to stay thin," she says.

Like many other teens, those with cystic fibrosis will also experiment with smoking. "That one drives me crazy, but there's no point saying 'Don't smoke.' Then they will. I say: 'How few smokes can you deal with in a day?' I try to get them to fix their own limit. Adolescence is a grey time, a time of experimentation, so you have to be grey with them, you have to be flexible," Gold says.

Another difficult ethical issue the nurse has to deal with is sexual activity among teens who are admitted to hospital for treatment.* "What if a girl has a boyfriend in the room and they are necking? We used to routinely kick them out and give them a lecture. But many of these guys are tremendously supportive. They can be a motivator in treatment, and really push them to take their meds and do their physio to stay healthy," Gold says.

The key to Gold's work is winning the trust of her patients (whom she often lovingly refers to as "my kids"). She knows that adherence to a treatment regime during the adolescent years has a

---

* If lung function decreases, CF patients are hospitalized and undergo therapy that consists of seven days of IV antibiotics, and aggressive physiotherapy.

major impact on how the disease will progress during adulthood. She knows, too, that if teens have even one adult they can talk to unencumbered—and it's rarely going to be an authority figure such as a parent or teacher—it can make a tremendous difference in their lives.

Despite medical advances, the life expectancy of males with CF is still only 32, and females 30, so teenagers with CF, more so than their peers, need someone to talk to frankly. They think about things that other adolescents don't. The fact that they're not going to get better is a tough issue. They have a constant awareness of their own mortality.

Gold's ability to discuss life-and-death issues with a volatile clientele, to do so with frankness and compassion, earned her the humanitarian award, the highest honour bestowed on staff members by the Hospital for Sick Children. (She was nominated by parents of kids with CF.) She says the children have given her more than she could ever give back. "They make me really appreciate my life in ways I never anticipated. They can teach you a lot about making the most of the time you have. They really teach you humility."

Just Like Granny—Catherine Bowness

There was a time, not so long ago, when, if your child fell ill, you would give your mother or grandmother a call, and the wise older woman—who almost certainly lived downstairs, or just down the street—would offer up an instant diagnosis and prescription for the ailment, which usually included a healthy dose of chicken soup.

But family life has changed dramatically in a couple of generations. Mother and grandmother are as likely as not to live thousands of kilometres away. Like you, they may well have been raised with ready access to doctors instead of a basket full of home remedies.

Calling a family physician at home in the middle of the night is now unheard of. And the prospect of sitting in an emergency room for six hours, or searching for a drop-in clinic with extended hours, is unappealing. But doing nothing, just waiting, is frightening, because of the remote but ever-present fear that what appears to be a routine childhood illness could actually be something serious.

So where do parents turn for practical advice about dealing with rashes, vomiting, headaches, nosebleeds, and the other ailments of daily life? A growing number of Canadians are reaching for the phone. Provinces, in response to consumer demand, and in a bid to cut emergency-room visits, are establishing telemedicine programs. Most of them are staffed by registered nurses such as Catherine Bowness.

"Grandmother might not be so handy anymore, so the telenurse becomes a substitute," says the telemedicine nurse at Clinidata in Moncton, New Brunswick. "Parents call about chicken pox, fever, diarrhea, the flu, all the things that you used to ask your grand-mother about."

Bowness is one of the growing number of nurses now working in private enterprise. Telehealth was initially a service offered by the regional health board, but later it was privatized. (Clinidata, which has a contract with the New Brunswick government to operate the telehealth service, is a division of a large communica-tions company called Oracle Assistance Group.) Nurses had to choose between retaining their seniority within the health board and finding another specialty, or sticking with telehealth and start-ing anew.

New Brunswick, the country's call-centre capital, has invested heavily in telemedicine, and the approach is paying big dividends. After only a few years, the hotline has become an integral part of the health system, and emergency-room visits have dropped dramatically. Of the 500 calls the service receives daily, only 13 per cent end up at Emergency. The vast majority are dealt with by a nurse on the phone—to the delight of most patients.

When a parent or patient calls the telehealth number, the call goes to a receptionist, who gets basic details (name, phone number) and does a quick screening (for example, emergency calls get transferred immediately to 9-1-1). The call is prioritized, and a nurse calls the patient back, usually within minutes.

When Bowness calls, she first checks that all demographic information is correct, then brings up the patient's medicare file on her computer screen. She asks basic, precautionary health-related questions: "Are you diabetic? Do you have high blood pressure? Any allergies?" Then she starts tackling the problem at hand.

About two-thirds of calls relate to pediatrics, so one of the parents is usually on the line, with the child nearby. "If the most obvious symptom is vomiting, I punch up 'vomiting' on my screen. Then I start the assessment: 'How many times in the last eight hours? Has he urinated? What's his temperature? How was the temperature checked? What's his colour like? What colour are his lips? What about his play activity?' That's an important indicator with children. 'Does he have any other symptoms like a rash?' "

Essentially, Bowness does the same thing as a nurse who does an initial assessment in the emergency room, except the caller acts as her eyes, ears, and hands. It is an assessment with only second-hand information. "Sometimes I feel like a blind emergency-room nurse," she says by way of analogy.

What Bowness needs, in lieu of the ability to see and touch, is an acute ability to listen and visualize. "You have to really develop your communications skills in this job. You ask a lot of questions, and you pick out the important things that people tell you. But you have to be careful how you do it: You don't want to lead them, you want them to tell you what's really happening, not what they think you want to hear."

Telemedicine nurses are not allowed to ad lib. The approach used is symptom-based, and nurses adhere to strict protocols, for medical and legal reasons. Practically speaking, that means that a caller should get the exact same diagnosis and advice if he calls with the same problem and speaks to three different nurses on three different occasions. Bowness, a senior nurse associate, will spend some of her time monitoring other calls to ensure that protocols are respected. But nurses also have input, recommending how the software (called

"Sharp Focus," it is imported from the United States) can be updated and modified.

The key role of the telemedicine nurse is to determine exactly what the problem is, and how it can be handled. The software provides them with a specific list of questions to determine if the child needs further treatment or if parents can take care of it alone.

Chicken pox, for example, is one of the illnesses easiest to diagnose over the phone because of the characteristic itchy rash and fluid-filled blisters. If the case is routine, the nurse tells the parent how to wash the child and how to spot infection. If the pox are large and encrusted, and the child has a high fever and is lethargic, the nurse instead urges parents to see a physician within twenty-four hours. In all cases, Bowness will guide callers through the illness, trying to educate them, and prepare them for what will happen next. She also encourages them to call back for anything, at any time. (Other telemedicine services, such as Quebec's Info-Santé, actually make a call-back an integral part of the nurse's routine.)

Calls take an average of about ten minutes, but range from a minute or so for a straightforward question to about half an hour for an elaborate problem. Bowness takes between thirty-two and forty calls per shift, and says they tend to flow in quite steadily. Flu season is, by far, the busiest. "But the challenge is to never prejudge. You have to listen to each story individually and never jump to conclusions," she says.

Each call is classified according to its disposition. There are four categories. "Handle at home" is the most common recommendation. A good portion of callers are urged to see a doctor within twenty-four hours, usually if they require a prescription. When a nurse urges a "see within two hours," it is because the illness or injury is serious, and would be better dealt with at a clinic or a doctor's office than by clogging up Emergency. Finally, there are a minority of calls that, despite what a caller said in his or her initial presentation, are truly emergencies.

"The truth is you never know how urgent a call will be. Denial is a big part of some illnesses, so sometimes callers withhold important information from the receptionist," Bowness says. For example, a caller might call about a "little nosebleed," and it turns out a child has been bleeding steadily from the nose for twenty-five minutes; another may talk about a bruise from a fall, and it turns out the child was unconscious for an undetermined length of time. People with chronic illnesses like cardiovascular disease might call about chest pains and suddenly find themselves having a heart attack or stroke. In those cases, the nurse will call an ambulance directly and stay on the line until it arrives, counselling other people on how to do first aid or cardiopulmonary resuscitation (CPR).

While there are many routine calls, about flu and chicken pox, for example, there are calls that the nurses find haunting. For Bowness, the most difficult are those where it is obvious child abuse is involved. Like all other medical professionals, nurses have an obligation to report those cases to the authorities. "We get calls from babysitters and daycares because they think the kids are being abused. Those cases really bother you." Also difficult to handle are suicide calls. While telehealth will try to refer callers to the local suicide hotline, there are many cases where the person appears in imminent danger and the nurse will remain on the line, doing counselling—again, according to protocol. "When I started this job, I would have this triage nightmare every night, and wake up in a cold sweat because every call was an emergency," Bowness recalls. "Now I sleep much better. I don't get calls in my sleep anymore."

In New Brunswick, telehealth doubles as the poison hotline, and Bowness says those calls can be among the most challenging. For example, a child who has been exposed to the fumes of fertilizer can be difficult to diagnose. The nurse may not know the type of fertilizer, or whether it is interacting with another chemical. Symptoms can change quite rapidly. "I find the poison calls make you nervous. In this job you always ask yourself: 'If I make a mistake, what will be the worst-case scenario for this caller tomorrow morning?' Then, you always err on the side of caution. If we have any doubts at all, we don't hesitate to send them to Emergency."

Clinidata is located in an office building in a nondescript industrial park. Bowness works in a small cubicle, wearing a telephone headset and continually reading data off the computer, or taking notes. While referring to the protocol, and chatting on the phone, she also fills in a nursing chart. The trick is doing the three seamlessly.

Bowness says some nurses are quite down on telemedicine, believing telenurses are so bound by protocols and computer programs that they lose their ability to do nursing. But Bowness, who has worked in emergency, intensive care, and a variety of roles in coronary care, sees telemedicine as a specialization like any other. She notes that nurses who assist in heart surgery have strict protocols, and no one would suggest they are robots. As with any type of nursing, the education and experience of the nurse are what make the protocols possible.

She cites the example of a parent who called for "general information" about circumcision. In passing, the caller talked about "discharge," and Bowness directed the conversation to the newborn. After more probing and prodding, it turned out the child had a green discharge that was unrelated to his recent circumcision, but that set off alarm bells about severe dehydration. The call, and the nurse's ability to read between the lines, probably saved the child's life. "You get a lot of calls like that, where people know something is wrong, but they don't know what it is, and they don't know how to articulate their concerns," she says. "If the child is in front of you, it's an easy diagnosis, but on the phone you have to be a lot more creative."

Bowness believes the care she provides is important precisely because it is so basic. "Sometimes parents call with really simple questions, like: 'Can I give my kid Tylenol?' For them, that question's really important and there's nowhere else to get an answer. I think that's why telehealth has become so popular."

Like a lot of nurses, Bowness always took it for granted that nurses worked in hospitals, and deliberated over the career move for a long time, particularly because her seniority ensured job security. So far, she hasn't seen a downside to working in private enterprise. The pay is slightly better than in hospitals. Raises are based on performance, not seniority. The hours are far better. Shifts are eight hours, and staggered to begin between 6:00 A.M. and 4:00 P.M. (The busiest times are early morning and early evening, the times of day when parents realize their kids are sick.)

Bowness says that, when she was working in a hospital, she would finish her shift physically and mentally exhausted, yet frustrated that she had not had an opportunity to sit and talk with any patients. Morale in her workplace is really good, something she never hears from hospital nurses anymore.

"As funny as it sounds, you can really develop a relationship with a patient on the phone. From a nursing perspective, that's very rewarding," Bowness explains. Ironically, people are turning to telemedicine to get the intimacy and personal touch they once expected in hospitals and at medical clinics. "Callers feel free to tell us everything. Maybe it's because they don't see us that it gives them the freedom to say things. And because they get our undivided attention—something you never get in a hospital anymore—people really feel we care. That's the one thing we hear over and over again: 'You guys really care.' "

Part Three
GROWING
INTO ADULTHOOD

The Tough Choices

In the first two years of life, a child undergoes a dramatic transformation in terms of development. A growth spurt of this magnitude, both physical and emotional, will occur at only one other time in a person's life—adolescence.

While there are hundreds of pediatric programs for newborns, the number of specialized adolescent-health programs in Canada remain few and far between. In fact, because teenagers tend to be healthy, they are routinely ignored by the medical system. This is a mistake.

During these formative years, teenagers make lifestyle choices involving nutrition, sexual responsibility, fitness, and drug and alcohol use that will have repercussions for the rest of their lives and, by extension, for the publicly funded health-care system.

It is a time in life when health promotion can have a dramatic impact—if campaigns are properly targeted, and carried out by professionals such as nurses.

In Part Three, you will meet Helen Thomas, a nurse-researcher and one of the country's leading experts in the field of determinants of health, the study of the connection between socio-economic conditions and health. Her views—that the single best way to improve the health of Canadians is by creating a national daycare program, and that most school-based health-education programs are a flop—are controversial and cutting-edge.

Thomas loves to work with teenagers, in large part because, like her, they continually challenge the system. She also feels they get a bad rap, and a raw deal from our health system, much the way public-health nurses do.

Despite the sex, drugs, and punk rock stereotype, most adolescents make responsible choices. The largest-ever survey of teenagers in Canada, conducted in 1999, found that the majority of youth do not have sex, smoke, drink, or fight.

Yet, when teens do take risks, they tend to take big risks. By Grade 12, three of every four students have still not had sexual intercourse. Among the minority who do have sex, more than 40 per cent said they do not use condoms, and 20 per cent do not use any birth control whatsoever.

Most youth actually become sexually active during their university or college years. Tammy Blackwell, a nurse at a university health clinic, deals with everything from broken hearts to broken limbs and, more to the point, with sexually transmitted diseases (STDs) and unwanted pregnancies.

Fifteen in every 1,000 young people have chlamydial infection. This can have serious implications down the road, particularly for women, because scarring increases the risk of ectopic pregnancies and infertility. Aside from STDs, more than 38,000 young women under the age of 20 become pregnant each year. Even in teenagers, childbirth is the single greatest reason for hospital admission in Canada. Teenage mothers, because they are at high risk for delivering low-birth-weight babies, are also a key clientele for public-health nurses.

Two out of every five teenagers terminate their pregnancies. You will also meet Suzane Fournier, a nurse in a Montreal abortion clinic. Because of overzealous anti-choice proponents, her job is one of the most dangerous in the nursing profession. Sex, and birth control in particular, is one of the most politically charged issues that nurses have to deal with, an area where they have been social trailblazers for decades.

Teenagers and young adults use the health-care system, but they tend to do so without continuity. Many pass up family physicians in favour of clinics that offer more anonymity, and do not require an appointment. Universities have done a good job of catering to this clientele and their needs. Many young people are looking for guidance and advice, and clinic nurses provide the sounding board they cannot find anywhere else.

The sad reality, however, is that the closest thing Canada has to a network of teen clinics is the country's emergency rooms and trauma centres. Karen Johnson is a nurse in the trauma ward of Sunnybrook and Women's College Health Sciences Centre, the country's busiest. She and her colleagues, who deal with the most severely injured patients in the health system, see more than their fair share of adolescents.

Risk-taking and adolescence are, at times, synonymous. The leading cause of death among teenagers is motor-vehicle accidents. For each one killed in such an accident, seventy-five are injured, often gravely. As well, teenagers like risky sports such as snowboarding, skateboarding, in-line skating, and snowmobiling, activities that result in many emergency-room visits. Each year, hundreds of healthy young people are wheeled into hospitals critically injured, and some sustain injuries that leave them paraplegic or quadriplegic.

Trauma nurses know better than anyone the value of public-health education. They know that only half of adolescents wear seat belts regularly, and more than one-third have driven a car while under the influence of alcohol or drugs.

Much is made of youth violence by the media. Almost 42 per cent of males and 18 per cent of females report having been in a physical fight during their high-school years. Nurses and teachers report that there are not more confrontations, but that they tend to be more violent. In emergency wards, knife wounds are commonplace, and gunshot wounds are no longer uncommon. (In the big teen survey, 1 per cent of students said they had carried a gun to school in the previous month.)

Canada does not think of itself as a violent country, but the third leading cause of death among teenage girls here is homicide.

Nonetheless, most teen violence is turned inward, as is evident from our epidemic of teen suicide. The average rate of suicide for children under the age of 14 in Canada is 2.2 per 100,000, up from 1.2 a decade ago; research by Statistics Canada shows that more than 8 per cent of teenage girls and 5 per cent of teenage boys have seriously considered taking their own lives.

Nurses who work with adolescents clearly deal with a volatile, challenging clientele. They work in a variety of settings, from high-tech trauma centres to local community centres. While they provide health care to the "healthy," these nurses can make a dramatic difference in the lives of their patients. They can also teach us a valuable lesson about the need to reform the public health-care system.

Thinking Upstream — Helen Thomas

When Helen Thomas was a nursing student at Toronto's Hospital for Sick Children in the early 1960s, it was an exciting time. She and other nurses were being trained to work with a new wave of high-technology equipment that would prolong and save the lives of many children. Yet at the same time, children, in particular, poor children, were still dying in large numbers from relatively common bacterial and viral infections.

"I remember quite distinctly saying one day: 'If kids are hungry, if they're getting sick because they're malnourished, why don't we nurses get out there and feed them instead of waiting for them to get sick and giving them IV fluids for gastroenteritis?' They just treated me like I was nuts," Thomas says today. "But we were using all this fancy technology to save their lives, and then, if we were successful, sending them back out there to conditions of poverty again. It didn't make much sense in 1964, and it makes even less sense today."

Decades later, Thomas's "nutty" ideas about improving population health through social rather than medical interventions are gaining mainstream acceptance. An associate professor of nursing at McMaster University, in Hamilton, she teaches a core course called "Health, Science and Society," and is one of the leading researchers in the field of determinants of health. Much of her work challenges traditional and conventional notions of how health is gained and lost, and, along with others,* Thomas is leading a so-called paradigm shift in health scholarship. What distinguishes her from her better-known counterparts, however, is that most of her research has a strong nursing component, and she has paid particular attention to adolescents, a group that is one of the most overlooked in the health-care system.

"The teenage group is the only one whose health has not improved in the last decade," Thomas points out. Their social and economic status has also worsened. The dropout rate, already at an appalling level, is up. So are teen pregnancies, and teen suicides. So, too, are sexually transmitted diseases, smoking, drinking, and virtually every other risk behaviour that has been measured. Yet, according to the medical model, teens are healthy.

As a clinical consultant to the Social and Public Health Services Division for the Region of Hamilton-Wentworth (she is on loan half-time by the university), Thomas does cutting-edge health research. For example, she conducted a detailed literature review of a whole range of school-based interventions directed at teenagers. The findings were shocking: The programs being used in schools are not very effective at all. The problem, Thomas says, is that most schools and school boards insist on schoolwide or districtwide programs, and young people have greatly varying levels of development and needs.

"We've got to find a new way of doing things if we want to improve the health of teenagers. We need programming targeted at level of risk, and we have to take into account gender in this age group too," she says. For example, girls who are sexually active with multiple partners get the same pregnancy-prevention message

* Notably Dr. Fraser Mustard, founder of the Canadian Institute for Advanced Research; Robert Evans, a health economist at the University of British Columbia; and Dan Offord, director of the Centre for Studies of Children at Risk.

as girls who are not sexually active, and the result is that neither group is served well. And, more alarmingly, Thomas has found that suicide-prevention programs may, in some instances, actually make boys more likely to commit suicide.

As part of a research project in the early 1990s, Thomas was asked to find solutions for a rural Ontario high school* that had a high number of marginalized students who were skipping classes and eventually dropping out. She recommended a nurse be put in the school to do teaching and see students one-on-one. The school nurse then helped establish a student health centre. "There's a lot of evidence in the literature that marginalized kids need to be brought into the mainstream. So, we took the principles of community development and let the kids run it, with a nurse in charge." The "losers" in school took charge, and established peer-counselling programs, and helped adapt the health- and sex-education curriculum. Empowered, they all started going to school again.

But, after almost four years, the school pulled the plug, and funding was lost. The short version of a long story is that, in an area where there are many Christian fundamentalists, the teenagers' demands for honest, straightforward sex education caused a tremendous backlash. "This program failed because it was so successful. The kids got assertive and demanding, they wanted programs tailored to them. That's something that huge bureaucracies like school boards really can't handle. They felt quite threatened," the nurse recalls.

Over the years, Thomas has developed strong views, often well ahead of her time. For example, she has been saying for years that the single most important thing we could do to improve the health of Canadians (particularly the poor) is to implement a national daycare program, a belief that is now gaining wide acceptance. "People know that this approach makes sense, but the reality makes them uncomfortable. With politicians, it's a lot worse. When people like me say health is related to poverty, they go

* Thomas asked that the school not be named because controversy over the project lingers.

crazy. They're willing to hear about cancer, but not poverty."

Not surprisingly, Thomas has butted heads repeatedly with those running the system, with everyone from politicians to health-and-welfare program administrators. What she has learned is that the public is more open-minded than its elected leaders, and that health programs are best delivered in the community, with the intimate involvement of those who will benefit from them. Increasingly, then, she has been moving into the field of community development.

When Thomas undertook a health-promotion project in East Hamilton, one the country's poorest neighbourhoods, the first thing done was a survey to find out what residents thought was good in their community, so there would be a basis from which to build. There was overwhelming interest in Warden Park, a big green space that the city was letting return to nature, so citizens decided to reclaim it. With a lot of hard work—much of it volunteer labour and lobbying—the park was transformed into a multiuse facility featuring sports fields and a beautiful playground. And, as a nurse, Thomas felt the exercise was a public-health success story. "Community development, like personal health, is an ongoing exercise in problem-solving. The women—and most of them were women—who tackled Warden Park became highly politicized; they learned how to set goals and achieve them. That translates into a healthier community and, eventually, into healthier residents," Thomas points out.

What academics like her are beginning to understand—and this is the basis of the determinants of health model—is that health is contextual more than it is cause-and-effect. "There is almost as much evidence today for social support in health as there was about the dangers of cigarettes when we started anti-tobacco campaigns. This is not speculation anymore, it's fact."

Yet, the biggest impediment to implementing programs that can have a dramatic long-term impact on the health of Canadians— and, by extension, on health-care costs—is the system itself. Governments tend to be organized in silos, and they budget in the short term, so long-term, across-the-board savings do not tend to pay political dividends.

Take, for example, an ongoing research project Thomas is overseeing using public-health nursing to reduce the incidence of child abuse. Recurrence rates range from 40 to 70 per cent a year, so, in the project, a family is assigned a nurse after a first abuse report, and she does two years of follow-up, including counselling on a range of health and parenting issues. The social-work approach has not been successful in breaking the pattern of violence and the hope is that nurses, by taking a different tack, will have more luck. "The 'problem' is that, if we're right, if we're successful, we won't save health-care dollars. Child abuse doesn't cost the health-care system much money. But, if you stop the cycle of violence, you will have an impact on the social-welfare, education, and criminal-justice systems. While that should be attractive, it's a hard sell," Thomas admits.

As a professor, Thomas often returns to her own experience as a student, when technology was less advanced. "You can go into a neonatal unit today and be more overwhelmed than I was forty years ago. It's truly amazing that these little peanuts will live. But equally important is realizing that low birth weight is the single most important determinant of health. They will live, but what kind of life will it be? And, once we wean them off the machines, what can we do as nurses to ensure their good health? It's not enough for us to produce excellent technicians. We have to teach nurses to think upstream," Thomas says.

She believes that nurses are in a unique position to change the health system, because they are the only health professionals who move rather seamlessly from institutions to the community. Thomas notes that one of the biggest single issues in our illness-care system is the lack of interface between institutions and the community. In many cases, nurses have made that transition; now they must help the system make the same shift.

Heartbreak and Beyond—Tammy Blackwell

Simon Fraser University (SFU) sits high atop Burnaby Mountain, a lush mecca for almost 20,000 students and staff. It is a privileged community: young, healthy, educated, and affluent.

For a health professional, it is a challenge caring for a population that is sexually adventurous, physically daring, emotionally volatile, and highly stressed.

"It's like a little city up here—the kind of city you really don't find anywhere else—and we're the local hospital," says Tammy Blackwell, a nurse at SFU Health Services. "We treat everything from the common cold to STDs [sexually transmitted diseases]. We do pap exams, treat sport injuries and workplace injuries, and deal with heart attacks. We even had a serious measles outbreak. It's a little bit of everything, but it's always on the cutting edge."

The clinic itself, located in the main student services building, is spacious and modern, with four exam rooms, a surgery room, and a cardiac room. It is staffed by four physicians (all of them salaried) and four registered nurses. With a mandate to offer continuous, easily available, high-quality health care, the clinic operates in a drop-in style, with few scheduled appointments.

Young women, who tend to be more acutely aware of their bodies and their health than are their male counterparts, use the clinic the most. Painful menstrual cramps, pap smears, and examinations for breast cancer are some of the most common reasons they make an appointment with a nurse. (And practice guidelines are being extended so nurses can conduct the pap test instead of a doctor doing it.) Young men, on the other hand, tend to come in for treatment of sports injuries and mental-health problems. The clinic also offers allergy shots and immunizations, including vaccines required for travel abroad.

But the predominant concerns for the clinic's clientele tend to be stress and sexual health. Birth control and safe-sex items, including the Pill and condoms, are made available free of charge to students. Still, there are a number of unplanned pregnancies each year. "I break the bad news to them a lot of the time. Young women with unwanted pregnancies, with cervical cancer. It's one of the toughest aspects of the job," Blackwell says. Nurses also do a lot of education work, both on a one-on-one basis, at the clinic, and in public forums, notably in university residences. Public education and counselling for women focus on eating disorders, and for men on steroid use.

Turn-out for sessions on sexual matters is always high, though women predominate. Blackwell says the level of knowledge is surprising. "Maybe I was naïve, but I didn't even know what an STD was until I went to nursing school. These kids have some pretty detailed questions." They also have a high incidence of sexually transmitted diseases. Blackwell says that, because the issue is highly publicized, most students are quite aware of HIV-AIDS, with many routinely getting tested before beginning a new sexual relationship. Gonorrhea and syphilis, once scourges among sexually active youth, are now rarely seen. But Blackwell says there has been a troubling increase in cases of herpes, genital warts, and chlamydia. Because of its young, hip clientele, the clinic is, in many ways, an early warning system of STD trends that will come to the general population. This is also true of social trends that have public-health repercussions, such as tattooing, the renewed popularity of hallucinogens, and a growing acceptance of prostitution. (In fact, the clinic now sees a number of students who work part-time as escorts to pay their way through school.)

While many STDs are readily treatable, or manageable, a diagnosis can provoke quite an emotional response, particularly in a young person who has always been healthy or to whom a partner has lied. "I think what makes us different from a private clinic is that we don't just treat the STD, we treat the heartbreak too," says Blackwell.

Another distressing issue that nurses at a university clinic increasingly have to deal with is date rape, in particular, victims of date-rape drugs.* While there is a sexual-assault centre on campus, clinic policy is to allow nurses to follow through with a victim as long as she desires, another example of the holistic approach they take to healing.

Mental-health issues are often handled by the clinic. Blackwell cites the example of a brilliant graduate student, newly married and "with everything going for her," who started to have all sorts of problems both in her personal life and in school. She came to the clinic for counselling, only to be diagnosed with severe manic depression. "The mental-health issues are definitely the hardest to deal with, because they are often diagnosed when people are in their early twenties. Lots of these kids are talented and gifted, and their lives get turned upside down," Blackwell notes. Addictions to drugs and alcohol also begin to reveal themselves in the university environment—with smoking heroin and ingesting so-called designer drugs two of the youth trends that are leading to problems.

Stress is one of the most widespread and devastating conditions the clinic has to deal with on a daily basis. By the time mid-terms roll around, it reaches epidemic proportions and pushes some students to the brink of suicide. "I think the biggest change I've seen over the years is stress levels. School is expensive, so most of them work jobs in addition to studying; the job market is tight, so they do outside activities to get on their résumés; and parents are really demanding, particularly those of Chinese students, and they are a big part of the population. There is so much pressure today, we could have a full-time stress clinic and never lack patients," Blackwell says. As a nurse, she spends much of her time teaching students coping mechanisms, such as time management and prioritizing tasks, and the importance of a balanced diet and regular exercise, "stuff that will help them not only through the crisis of mid-terms, but their whole lives."

Because Simon Fraser is such an isolated site, clinic nurses also

* At present, there are two principal date-rape drugs, Rohypnol, a prescription drug and sedative ten times stronger than Valium, and GHB (gamma-hydroxy-butyrate), a depressant that can be easily manufactured in a home laboratory.

serve a paramedic role on campus, and they are trained in advanced cardiac life-support. When a worker fell off the roof of a building, Blackwell helped stabilize the patient until an ambulance could arrive—it takes a minimum of thirteen minutes for an emergency vehicle to get up the hill after a 9-1-1 call—and transport him to a trauma centre. As there would be in any small town, there are also broken bones from falls, epileptic seizures, and a few cardiac incidents at SFU each year.

Physically, the most demanding part of the nurses' role is getting to the scene of these emergencies. The medical equipment Blackwell carries to an emergency, including a defibrilator, weighs more than 20 kilograms; because of the many stairs, it gets slung over her shoulder.

But Blackwell would not trade the job for a return to the hospital. "It's so much fun working with students. They're generally healthy and they always have a sense of humour. They're not complainers at all, and they respond really well to treatment and counselling." The hours, 8:30 A.M. to 5:30 P.M. daily—no nights, no weekends—are also a big attraction. "The pay is crappy compared to a hospital, but the hours almost make up for it," she points out. "You get so much variety here: You're a public-health nurse, educator, emergency technician—all rolled into one. You never, ever get bored with your work."

A Question of Choice—Suzane Fournier

About 110,000 abortions are performed in Canada annually. There are few medical procedures that are more common, fewer still that are less complex. The procedure takes about three minutes, requiring no more than a local anaesthetic and a mild painkiller. A woman can choose to terminate a pregnancy, walk into an abortion clinic, and walk out again in a couple of hours.

"Abortion is legal, it's safe and it's straightforward. But it's still taboo in our society, so women come with a lot of baggage," says Suzane Fournier, a nurse at the Morgentaler Clinic in Montreal.

"Abortion is a lot more than a medical procedure; it's an intensely personal choice for a woman."

As they do in most specialties, nurses at the clinic have two distinct facets to their jobs: technical and patient support. Fournier says that less than 25 per cent of her time is relegated to the former. "Our philosophy is to be woman-centred, not act-centred, so my primary concern is always the client."

In most major cities, a woman seeking to terminate a pregnancy need look no further than "abortion" in the Yellow Pages. Most hospitals perform abortions at no cost. It is a basic health service that has been legal, and without restriction, since the abortion law was struck down by the Supreme Court of Canada in 1988.* Not-for-profit and for-profit clinics charge between $150 and $600, depending on the number of weeks of pregnancy. The routine is similar at most clinics.

A woman gets basic information over the phone. "The first two questions are always 'Does it hurt?' and 'How much does it cost?' " says Fournier. At the Morgentaler Clinic, that initial call is usually fielded by a clerical worker, though sometimes by a nurse. The woman is asked whether she has taken a pregnancy test, and when her last menstrual cycle was. (Abortions are generally not performed under five weeks because the cervix is still too firm.) Appointments can usually be booked within days at clinics, though it can take six weeks at a hospital. (Hospital gynecologists do not like to perform the procedure because it pays poorly, so there are lengthy waiting lists.)

When a woman arrives for an appointment, she first meets a counsellor. At the Morgentaler Clinic, the counsellor happens to be a sex therapist. There is a medical questionnaire, with emphasis on gynecological history. Then the counsellor meets the woman alone; afterwards, if she chooses, she and her partner can have a

* Prior to that time, therapeutic abortions could only be performed legally in a hospital, following approval by a committee of three doctors, a process the highest court deemed to be arbitrary, demeaning, and potentially injurious. A number of family doctors such as Dr. Henry Morgentaler, however, performed abortions for a number of years before the ruling.

counselling session. "There is no good or bad reason for an abortion. We don't judge women. Our primary concern is that the decision is the woman's own, and that it is sound. We don't want a woman to be there because she is being coerced, or based on gross misinformation—say, she wants a baby but has taken one aspirin and is afraid of birth defects," Fournier says. "We often hear women say 'I have no choice.' That's not an answer. We try to help them understand that choice can be agonizing, it can be painful, but it's a choice, one that belongs to them alone."

If the woman chooses to proceed—and the policy at the Morgentaler Clinic is that a client can back out at any moment without incurring any cost—the nurse takes over. First, there is an ultrasound. This is a crucial step—particularly psychologically. "After a positive pregnancy test, most women have this mental image in their head of a fully formed baby. At seven weeks, the embryo measures half a centimetre. The ultrasound gives them a better grounding in the reality," Fournier says.

The ultrasound takes ten to twenty minutes. Once again, the technical aspect is swift, but women take the opportunity to talk with the nurse. "What you realize after years of doing this work is that the abortion is the easy part. Most women make that decision relatively easily. But being pregnant often forces a woman to re-examine her life, her relationship. It can be an emotional upheaval, not because it's an ethical dilemma or a painful medical procedure, but because it is a catalyst for putting your life and your feelings under a microscope," Fournier says.

The ultrasound is important not only for the woman, but for the doctor carrying out the procedure. Doctors are working blind, so the ultrasound locates the fetus and, for second-trimester abortions, provides a measurement for the fetus, particularly the head.

The next step is the abortion room. It is sparsely furnished, containing only a gynecological table and a chair (many women are accompanied during the procedure, though usually by a girlfriend or mother, rarely by a male partner). Again, there is time for questions for the nurse. She then tells the doctor when to enter.

The doctor first discusses birth-control options with the woman, and does routine screening for chlamydia and other sexually transmitted diseases. There is an educational aspect, but the approach is also designed to relax the woman. The nurse will administer painkiller intravenously, according to the client's wishes. There is more discomfort than pain, says Fournier, who likens the feeling of the procedure to menstrual cramps.

For pregnancies from five to fifteen weeks, the abortion procedure is identical—"manual vacuum aspiration" is the technical term. The doctor treats the cervix with a local anaesthetic (hormones excreted during pregnancy make it malleable), then there are three steps—dilatation (with a speculum), aspiration, and curettage—each of which takes about a minute. The process removes the fetus, placenta, and amniotic fluids. "During the intervention itself, the nurse's role is to provide support, answer the woman's questions, and provide more pain relief if necessary," Fournier says.

With late-term abortions—twenty weeks is the maximum at the Morgentaler Clinic—the process is more complex. The fetus must be extracted manually, and often it is sectioned in utero to facilitate that procedure. One of the nurse's roles is to ensure the extraction is complete. Fournier says that, in that regard, there is no difference between her work and that of nurses who work in childbirth, oncology, transplants, and amputations. "Medical professionals deal with all sorts of procedures that the general public finds gruesome, but they tend to get emotional only about abortion. After many years of working in labour and delivery, I can tell you that, in terms of what you see and hear, this work is no more difficult," she says.

The nurse, who has been confronted with the ethical issues surrounding abortion countless times over the years, responds to religious arguments with candour and confidence. "If you ask me, 'Does a fetus have a soul?' my answer is this: 'I have my beliefs, and they are firmly held beliefs. But as a nurse I have a responsibility towards the client, and an obligation to respect her choice that supersedes my personal views. I do not have the right to impose my beliefs on anyone, but I have an obligation to provide the best care possible to everyone,'" Fournier says.

Obviously, though, she has chosen to work in an abortion clinic. After twelve years of working in labour and delivery in a suburban Montreal hospital, Fournier saw an advertisement for a "feminist" nurse to work at a women's health clinic, Le Centre de santé des femmes. The downtown Montreal clinic provides birth-control counselling and abortions. "Until I went for a job interview, I had never really asked myself if I was pro-choice. Professionally, it just seemed like a natural evolution to me. Pregnancy and abortion to me are two sides of the same coin, two aspects of womanhood. It's a choice that most women have to make at some point in their lives: abortion or childbirth. And, you know, I don't question a woman's choice to have an abortion any more than I ever questioned a woman's choice to have a baby. As a nurse, why would I?" Fournier asks.

The Morgentaler Clinic in Montreal performs about 2,500 abortions annually. It is open four half-days, one night, and all day on Fridays (by far the busiest day). Summer is the busiest time, not because there are more abortions, but because many hospitals close their abortion services to save money. At private abortion clinics, the tensest time is fall, in particular the days surrounding Remembrance Day, when anti-choice zealots intensify their picketing, and when most shootings and bombings are carried out.*

The Morgentaler Clinic in Montreal is located in a medical office building in Montreal's trendy Plateau district. Unlike most clinics, it rarely sees picketers—Quebec was the first province to have a free-standing clinic, and public opinion has always been far more liberal here than elsewhere in the country. But the clinic does have all the amenities: a security camera, intercom system, bullet-proof

* In 1992, the Morgentaler Clinic in Toronto was bombed. It was closed at the time and no one was hurt. But a number of nurses and doctors working in U.S. abortion clinics have been killed.

windows, a bullet-proof metal door separating the waiting room and the abortion rooms, and panic buttons in every room.

Given the context, Fournier is surprisingly cavalier about the dangers of her line of work. "I feel I'm a lot less at risk than nurses who work in emergency rooms or psychiatric institutions. There is no predicting these things, and there is no point worrying. Look at the women at Polytechnique.* They probably thought they were in the safest place in the world, a university campus, and look at what happened," she says.

Like many women, Fournier knows from her own experience the importance of having safe, legal, easily accessible abortions. "Twenty years ago, when I needed an abortion, we only talked about these things in hushed voices, as if we should be ashamed of our choices as women. I was a nurse working in gynecology and I had no idea where you went for an abortion. Can you imagine how frightening it was for women in the general public who were denied even the ability to make a choice?" she asks. (When Fournier found a doctor, the soonest she could get an appointment was six weeks hence and, in the interim, she had a miscarriage. But the experience prompted her to learn more, and eventually influenced her career choice.)

As a nurse providing such a basic, necessary service, however, she finds it paradoxical to be working in the private sector. And doubly so because she is convinced that the service in clinics is far superior to that provided in hospitals. (About one-third of abortions are performed in clinics and two-thirds in hospitals.) In a city like Montreal, unless they are financially desperate, women will go to a private clinic, because waits are shorter, and the care more personal.

In Quebec, abortion is deemed to be a basic service, but that means only that at least one institution in each district must offer the service free of charge, not that it is covered universally. The fact that, in the twenty-first century, women are paying for abortions when so many other procedures, often less necessary, are covered

* On December 6, 1989, a feminist-hating gunman killed 14 women at l'École Polytechnique, an engineering school in Montreal. Most of the women were in class or in the cafeteria.

rankles Fournier. "That women have to pay for such a basic service disturbs me greatly. It reflects poorly on our public-health system and it's something that, as nurses, we should not tolerate."

The Golden Hour—Karen Johnson

There is, believe it or not, a trauma season. It runs from Victoria Day (nurses call it the "May Two-Four weekend") through to Thanksgiving, in October. During that period, there is a lethal mixture of more cars on the road and more beer coursing through the veins of young men.* Activity peaks markedly each Friday and Saturday, the party nights, when stabbings, shootings,† and gruesome sporting injuries get added to the mix.

"The approach we take is that we have one hour from the time of injury to save a patient's life. We call it the 'Golden Hour,' " says Karen Johnson, a trauma nurse and educator at Sunnybrook and Women's College Health Sciences Centre in Toronto. Forget what you have seen on the television program *ER*. What takes place after the ambulance or helicopter arrives is a well-choreographed medical ballet in which nurses play a starring role.

"For me, trauma nursing is the epitome of what I want to do in the profession. People do look at us as the be-all and end-all of nursing, but I don't think it's fair to rate it that way. We're really just another specialty in a profession that's becoming increasingly specialized, but we get a lot of attention because what we do is dramatic and spectacular," Johnson says.

There is usually two to ten minutes' notice before a patient arrives (extending to two hours' notice when a patient is transferred from elsewhere in the province). Only the most severely injured go to Sunnybrook, which deals with two-thirds of traumas in Ontario. During that time, nurses get their assignments, and a

* Sixty-one per cent of traumas involve motor-vehicle accidents. One-third of all trauma patients consumed alcohol in the hours prior to the accident, including half of all severely injured drivers.
† Stabbings and shootings account for one of every eight trauma cases.

briefing about the patient, and they start preparing for action.

There are ten people on each trauma team: three nurses, five physicians (a team leader, orthopaedic surgeon, neurosurgeon, general surgeon, and anaesthesiologist), and two technicians (an X-ray tech and a respiratory therapist). Each room is fully equipped with its own ultrasound, X-ray machine, and blood fridge, and can be used for emergency surgery. The trauma unit operates twenty-four hours a day, seven days a week. It is one of the most dramatic and expensive areas of the health-care system: cases cost an average of $18,000 during the few hours of intensive treatment they receive.

Nurse 1, the primary nurse, receives the initial report, records the history of the incident, documents treatment in the field or other facility, and briefs her colleagues. Once the patient arrives, she assigns the case an identification number and takes vital signs. Nurse 1 will stay at the patient's side through to disposition. She does all the charting, prepares all medications, labels all lab specimens, and enters the information into a computer. She is responsible for collecting clothes and valuables, and bagging them for evidence. (Many trauma cases involve criminal activity, from drunk driving to attempted murder.) Nurse 1 also goes everywhere with the patient, including when the patient goes for computed tomography (CT) scans and angiograms,* processes that can take up to five hours to complete. She will leave only when the patient has been delivered to the operating room (where two-thirds go), the intensive-care unit, or the morgue.

The primary nurse will also have dealings with the family along the way, to offer emotional support. "If you sense that a patient won't make it, you want the family in there while the heart is still beating. If you can give them five minutes to say some last words, that is valuable time, it means a lot," Johnson says.

* CT scans are a method of examining the body's soft tissues using X-rays. In trauma, the procedure is important for detecting dangerous fluid build-up.

Angiograms are a set of X-rays taken following the injection of a special liquid. They can show the condition of an artery to determine, for example, if it was damaged by a knife or bullet.

Nurse 2 is the circulating nurse. She does the initial survey of the trauma that will help determine the course of treatment and priorities, and initiates life-saving measures, alongside the physician. The four-pronged assessment is dubbed "ABCD": "A" for clearing the airway; "B" for checking breathing; "C" for determining circulation; and "D" for testing for disability or neurological damage. In trauma, every patient is assumed to have a spinal-cord injury until it is proven otherwise, so Nurse 2 ensures the spine is immobilized.

Because trauma patients tend to need large quantities of fluids and blood products, they get two intravenous lines, and Nurse 2 is responsible for hanging the bags. She hooks the patient up to the battery of high-tech monitors (cardiac, oxygen saturation, blood pressure). There are established protocols for procedures, but, essentially, a nurse can insert oral and nasal tubes, use a bag-valve mask, and establish oxygen, but not set up a ventilator.

Nurse 3 is also a circulating nurse. She does continual reassessments of the patient's condition and watches the monitors. Each fundamental body function—breathing, circulation, brain activity—is monitored on a cycle that can vary from thirty seconds to one hour. Nurse 3 also hangs all medication given intravenously, keeps track of all fluids, and marks bags. (Each drug and blood product can be traced back to a patient electronically.) As a patient stabilizes, the second circulating nurse will withdraw and move on to another case. Aside from those roles, about half of the trauma nurses also fly, either on the hospital's helicopter, *Bandage One*, or on medical evacuation flights.

Trauma, of course, is unpredictable. When it is quiet, nurses will help out with intensive-care and emergency patients. (The difference between "trauma" and "emergency" is that trauma involves severe, life-threatening injury, such as head injuries, spinal-cord damage, multiple fractures, or internal-organ damage.) But it can also get very busy.

There are about 800 trauma cases admitted to Sunnybrook annually, but Johnson has seen up to eight in a single shift, a dizzying pace. Technological advances and skills development mean that an astounding 88 per cent of those who come through the door—all with horrific injuries—actually survive. Many are literally brought back to life by the trauma team.

Opened in 1979, Sunnybrook's trauma unit is recognized as one of the best in the world. As such, it attracts some of the most talented nurses, including many it has wooed back home from the United States. They are expected to continually upgrade their qualifications, and Karen Johnson's role is to provide that educational component.

"You never see a nurse educator on *ER* because it's not a sexy job, but it's essential," she says. "What makes a good trauma nurse is the ability to make critical decisions. To do that, you have to be sharp, you have to be on top of your game, and the way to do that is education."

Johnson has been studying for more than ten years straight, trying, she says, to stay one step ahead of the nurses she teaches. Her job description is nineteen pages long, single-spaced. She does recertification of nursing staff, teaches new emergency-room protocols and techniques, prepares education manuals, assists in hiring, does orientation for new employees, is responsible for students, sits on a number of hospital committees, and facilitates research projects. There are seventy-five nurses on the unit, plus support staff, but her job is only a 0.7 position—meaning she is paid only 70 per cent of a full-time salary. Johnson also teaches at Centennial College.

She says one of the biggest failings of the Canadian health-care system is the lack of support for education. The shifting of ever-growing costs to nurses themselves in a public-health system is perverse, particularly at a time when big business is realizing the long-term benefits of investing in training and skills upgrades. "Getting nurses to pay for further education is a false economy. If you want to ensure the best possible care, the system should subsidize education, like they do in the United States," Johnson says. (In fact, one of the major attractions of nursing south of the border is the willingness of institutions to pay for courses, which can add up to thousands of dollars annually for a specialized nurse.) Sunnybrook nurses can apply for grants, but they cover only a fraction of tuition, and the hospital created Johnson's position as a way of providing some education free of charge.

Another area where the system fails nurses is in dealing with the traumatic events in trauma. Johnson says that burly, tough police officers, firefighters, and ambulance technicians have routine debriefings and access to psychologists to help them deal with the horrors they witness. Nurses, on the other hand, are left to their own devices.

"A couple of years ago, we had a nine-year-old drowning victim. He had been out twenty minutes in the field, so there wasn't much hope, but we really tried. I looked down at him on the bed and it was like looking at my own son. The physician said: 'Is everybody okay with calling it?' We all said okay, but then we fell apart one by one. Before we could even catch our breath, they were rolling in an MI [myocardial infarction, or heart attack, patient]. I didn't even have five minutes for a cry. But I still see that child's face every single day," says Johnson.

Johnson points out that trauma nurses are very supportive of each other, but going into a back room and talking it out is sometimes not enough. "But, unfortunately, the show must go on. The patients just keep rolling through the door." The saving grace is that most trauma nurses get an adrenaline rush each time an ambulance pulls up, and that allows them to keep doing the demanding job day after day. "Something keeps us here and it's definitely not the money. My father always said that nurses are born, not made. Maybe he was right."

Part Four
THE ADULT YEARS

Modern Wisdom

As you move into your thirties, forties, and fifties, the aches, pains, and stresses of daily life start to catch up with you. You may need elective surgery for minor woes. Indigestion may be mistaken for a heart attack. A polyp may be viewed as a sign of cancer. It may be time for a change of job, voluntary or otherwise. Dealing with the children now that they are becoming teenagers may be more trouble than you ever imagined. Your marriage may be shaky, and your finances shakier.

It is getting increasingly difficult to know where to turn for help with these important issues that can affect your health. Politicians and health-system administrators are quick to call on the public to take more responsibility for their health, but rarely do they provide the tools, or the ready access to information and advice, that are essential to doing so.

A good family physician, once the primary point of entry into the health-care system, is hard to find, and even then you are lucky to get fifteen minutes of his or her time. Provinces with community health clinics, such as Quebec with its CLSCs, make it a lot easier to access information and counselling. You can walk into a CLSC without an appointment and usually see a nurse (and, if necessary, a doctor) within an hour. They can deal with minor problems like wart removal or blood-pressure monitoring on the spot. They can also provide advice on diets and fitness, or referrals to specialists if there is a basis for more serious concern. But public clinics are also feeling the strains of underfunding.

Because most Canadians don't know where to turn, they tend not to seek advice on preventive health measures. Rather, they wait until they feel sick enough to get help, and then they end up in hospital emergency rooms. Studies routinely show that at least three-quarters of people who go into the emergency room are non-urgent cases. They should be getting treatment elsewhere, at a physician's office or a clinic.

Yet, by law, emergency rooms cannot turn people away. That places tremendous stress on emergency-room nurses, particularly those in the front lines. Barbara Harris, a veteran triage nurse, tells of the challenge of assessing dozens of patients each night. As people present themselves with everything from chest pains to hangnails, it is the nurse who must decide priority treatment. She also has to take the bulk of abuse doled out by those angry at the wait—invariably those with minor ailments who see others pass them by in the queue.

Harris's expertise in a particular area is typical of the approach of a growing number of nurses today. Clearly, the trend is towards specialization. This section features not only a triage nurse, but a burn nurse, two neurology nurses, a rheumatology nurse, and a public-health nurse who promotes quitting smoking. These are all jobs that did not exist a generation ago.

One condition that always gets top priority in emergency rooms is severe burns. In larger centres, those who suffer electrocution, chemical burns, or the ravages of flames bypass the trauma centre and go to a specialized burn unit. Working on this unit is one of the most demanding jobs in the profession because nurses will be assigned to a patient as soon as he arrives in critical condition, and remain with him throughout treatment, which can take a year. Anthony Arsenault, a burn nurse, has made the gut-wrenching journey with his patients many times.

Wendy Morrison is another kind of specialist, working in the

rapidly evolving field of neurology. She is also a researcher who
has had a hand in testing some of the most dramatic pharmaceutical advances in the field of treatment for multiple sclerosis (MS).
Nurses, particularly those with experience charting cases meticulously and dealing with ethical dilemmas, are much sought after in
research. With drug trials costing millions of dollars and the
potential for profits many times greater, drug manufacturers
cannot afford to have their research fall apart, and the coordina-
tion and communication skills of nurses such as Morrison have
proved invaluable.

Putting those discoveries to practical use is another role of
nurses. Thanks to medical advances, many more patients are living
much longer with chronic illnesses, and the health system has
struggled to find the most efficient way of dealing with them. The
result has been the creation of clinics where patients can get
specialized care.

It is not unusual today for large hospitals to have dozens of
these clinics, with a core of specialized nurses and physicians.
Nurses are the backbone of these clinics, as they are throughout
the health system. Two nurses who work in this setting are
Colleen Harris, a nurse-practitioner at a MS clinic in Calgary,
and Cheryl Magnusson, who works in an arthritis and lupus
clinic in Vancouver.

Patients not only make regular visits to clinics, but they can turn
to those nurses in a time of need and be assured of getting straight
answers from a health professional who knows the details of their
particular condition, as well as their personal story. This is important because chronic-disease management often has less to do with
the symptoms of a disease itself than with its impact on the
sufferer's job, relationships, and sex life. Harris has been seeing
some of her patients for more than a decade, which allows her to
speak frankly and to be far more perceptive when it comes to
seemingly unrelated issues that can have a significant impact on
patient health. Similarly, Magnusson, whose clientele is largely
women (many of whom are of child-bearing age but unable to

have children),* does more counselling than traditional medical care. But this is precisely what consumers have been saying for years—that they want to be active participants in their health care, not passive recipients of drugs and surgery.

No look at adult health would be complete without an examination of smoking, a habit that is shared by one-third of Canadians. Smoking kills more than 50,000 people annually in this country— more people than are killed by motor vehicle accidents, AIDS, suicide, and murder combined. Carol McDonald, a public-health nurse in Ottawa, has dedicated many years of her career to fighting the evils of tobacco, and she has proved to be a formidable foe.

Smoking is not the only problem that catches up to people as they start to age. Two-thirds of Canadians aged 45 to 64 are over-weight, and almost as many are inactive. The combination of cigarettes, poor diet, and lack of exercise is a recipe for poor health. The results are predictable, but the death and illness that occur are also largely preventable.

Nurses like McDonald have proven over the years that investing in public-health measures such as smoking cessation can have an appreciable impact. It is no coincidence that Ottawa–Carleton, which has the most aggressive anti-smoking measures in the country, also has the lowest smoking rates. Nurses could make a similar contribution in areas such as weight reduction and promotion of physical fitness. Yet the health system continues to spend, without limitation, on treatment, and remains miserly when it comes to investing in prevention.

Enlightened employers, on the other hand, recognize the value of prevention, understanding that healthy workers are more productive. An in-house clinic, usually staffed by an occupational-health nurse, is their solution. Lynda Kushnir Pekrul works as a nurse for a large insurance company. She speaks eloquently of the benefits of such a service, of providing care and counselling to employees who are dealing with modern issues such as infertility,

* Treatment is similar to chemotherapy and can damage the fetus.

caregiver stress, ulcers, weight control, and depression. Ironically, it is the private sector that has seen the cost-effectiveness of making occupational-health nurses readily available to the public, knowing that they can help avert major problems, and expenses, not far down the road.

The Walking Wounded — Barbara Harris

It's Friday, a crisp early winter's night in St. John's. The season's first snow has fallen, followed by freezing rain, and a thick blanket of fog has rolled in to create an eerie, horror-movie landscape. The emergency room is already crowded with the victims of traffic accidents, falls, and shovelling-induced back pains. As the evening wears on, the casualties of George Street stumble in faster than the earlier patients can be discharged: a patron who thinks he broke his arm when he slipped while leaving a bar; another whose nose was bloodied in a drunken fight, and who is struggling to stay awake; and a giggling student whose girlfriend is concerned about his consumption of beer with Ecstasy.* They are, in turn, greeted by the same nurse, who questions them crisply while jotting down notes. When she sits down for a second at the counter, a man clutching his back shuffles over to ask the same question for about the tenth time in the past ten minutes. She stares icily, answers "Soon," and calls someone else's name. The man swears loudly, and many of the others in the waiting room look away, rechecking the clock.

"Those nurses sitting there at the desk are not that popular, that's for sure," says Barbara Harris, division manager of Emergency at the General site of the Healthcare Corporation of St. John's, Newfoundland, with a mixture of laughter and exasperation. "But the perception that they are doing nothing is very wrong. The triage nurse is a key player on the emerg team. She is responsible for everyone in the waiting area, and she makes sure the patients flow

---

* "Ecstasy" is a club drug that depletes serotonin in the brain, causing euphoria and having a potentially dangerous effect on the heart. Its scientific name is methylene dioxymethamphetamine (MDMA).

through in a sensible manner, to make sure the right patients are seen first."

There are hundreds of hospital emergency rooms across Canada. Mention the hit television show *ER* to any nurse working in them and you will invariably elicit groans. Rare is the patient who stumbles to the counter clutching his chest from a knife wound. Rarer still is the patient who comes flying through the door on a gurney, accompanied by screaming paramedics and surrounded by a team of doctors.

The mundane reality is that most people walk into emergency rooms under their own volition, and the vast majority of them have a condition that does not require emergency treatment. "At the General site, about 75 to 80 per cent of our patients are non-urgent. That's around the national average, even a little low, because we handle trauma and a lot of other hospitals don't," Harris says. Dog bites are more common than gunshot wounds. Sprained ankles far more likely than stab wounds. Patients with rashes are more numerous than those with heart conditions. And those with sniffles from colds appear more frequently than victims of serious car crashes.

What they all have in common is that the first person they see when entering the emergency room is the triage nurse, a job that Harris has done for the better part of three decades. The initial assessment takes two or three minutes. Most patients think they are just chatting with a nurse, but she is processing their words and actions with all five senses. "Say, someone comes in with a sore stomach. It can be any number of things. So you start looking for clues: Is he doubled over in pain? Is he sweaty? What's his colour like? What kinds of symptoms does he have? Vomiting? Diarrhea? For how long? You ask about the pain, on a scale of one to ten. While you're talking, you're probably taking the pulse, maybe reaching for a wheelchair. There's a lot of things going on at the same time. You can do a whole assessment and the patient thinks nothing has happened yet because he hasn't seen a doctor," Harris says.

This initial assessment usually takes place even before registration (in some hospitals, the triage nurse does registration, while others use support staff). Even the most seemingly straightforward cases are seen within ten minutes. If there is a golden rule for a triage nurse, Harris believes, it is to assume nothing, to treat every case as potentially serious. "In triage, we have a lot of little sayings that we repeat in our heads: 'What you see is not always what you get,' 'All who stumble are not drunks,' 'Never assume an accident caused a condition,' and so on. They are just reminders that you can never take anything for granted."

Harris cites the example of a middle-age man, smelling heavily of liquor, who comes in for stitches after cutting his head in a fall. He seems okay, though a bit confused. The nurse cannot focus on the obvious wound, the small cut. Perhaps he has a concussion. Further, she cannot assume he fell because he drank too much. "In that case, it turned out the man's pacemaker malfunctioned. He fell because of a heart condition. It turns out he was not just a stumbling drunk, that he had quite a serious condition—priority one," she says. "In the emergency room, the burden is on the triage nurse to show it's not an emergency."

The fact that many people present themselves at Emergency with minor ailments does not make that easier. Trauma cases, on the other hand, are easy to triage. But differentiating chest pain due to indigestion from chest pain due to angina, or distinguishing between a headache from a hangover and one from an aneurysm, is not that simple, particularly when there are complicating factors, such as substance abuse or unrelated wounds from injuries, that make triage more difficult.

What is important to understand—and is largely misunderstood—is that the role of the nurse is not to diagnose, it is to determine what should happen next. In other words, to know enough to figure out how long a person can safely wait for diagnosis and treatment. Experience and intuition help, but the most important skill is critical thinking. Like many nurses, Harris is overly modest about her skills. She was part of a national team of nurses and physicians who formulated the emergency-department triage and acuity scale, a means of standardizing the manner in which patients are sorted.

Each patient is assigned a triage level, with 1 being the highest priority and 5 the lowest. The category indicates how quickly the patient needs to be seen, and by whom. A Level 1 is someone with a code (meaning the heart has stopped) or who is unresponsive, perhaps after a motor-vehicle accident or a stroke; such patients should see a nurse and a physician immediately. A Level 2 is conscious but has an emergent condition (one that could quickly grow far worse), such as a head injury, respiratory distress, or pain that is high on the scale; these patients should see a nurse immediately and a doctor within fifteen minutes. A Level 3 is injured but alert, with a pain scale ranking of 5–6; these patients are still considered urgent, and should see a nurse immediately and a physician within thirty minutes. A Level 4 is less urgent, say, a broken leg without any vascular injury; such patients should be seen within one hour. A Level 5 is a non-urgent case, such as a sore throat or an injury that is low on the pain scale; they should be seen within two hours, at least theoretically.

The triage nurse assigns these numeric rankings to each patient, and emergency-room nurses and physicians see them according to this assigned priority. Some larger hospitals have electronic tracking boards that ensure all high-priority patients get seen first but that, for example, a Level 5 patient who has been waiting five hours would be seen before a newly arrived Level 4. Others, like the General, have a handwritten flow board and trust the triage nurse to make the necessary adjustments.

The categorization of patients is not static. As she sits at the desk (something that rankles those who are waiting more than anything else does), the nurse not only has paperwork to do, but continually scans the room and reassesses patients visually. Patients are urged to return to the desk if their condition changes, and the nurse will often go into the waiting room to re-evaluate. "I think what most members of the public don't understand is that the

triage nurse is not just a policeman keeping them out of the treatment rooms. She really is taking care of them," Harris says.

As a long-time emergency-room nurse, she empathizes with the
frustrations of patients who have long waits, but wishes they
would step back and look at the big picture the way a triage nurse
is forced to do every minute of her shift. "I'm tempted to take
people in sometimes and show them some chest work, to show
them what a real emergency looks like. We don't keep them waiting just for the fun of it," Harris says.*

It is frustrating for emergency-room nurses to deal with a lot of
minor cases. They know better than anyone else that treating the
flu and acne in the emergency room is inefficient and expensive.
They also know that patients with the most trivial ailments are
invariably the most obnoxious.

"We get yelled at a lot, and I can't think of many instances
where it's justified," Harris says. "The toughest thing to take is,
right after a death, ... [being] confronted by someone yelling about
a broken toe, or something we can really do nothing about."
Harris says, diplomatically, that "we have to be very special
people then. Every triage nurse has to count to ten a lot in a shift."

But what about the perception that those who make a fuss get
treated faster? It's not really true. Everyone is assessed in the
same way. Loud people may get special attention, but not of a
medical kind. Emergency rooms in most hospitals now have
security guards, even police, on duty. Where the perception of
special treatment comes from is that people who are creating a
disturbance—especially those with psychiatric problems and
those who are drunk—will often be whisked off to a separate
room. But, usually, they are sent to an empty examining room,
and wait just as long as they would otherwise, though without
bothering other patients.

* A 1999 poll conducted by the consulting company PricewaterhouseCooper
showed that, in fact, most patients are satisfied with waiting times in Emergency.
Three-quarters of patients wait less than an hour, and one in five actually is
treated within fifteen minutes of arrival. Fewer than one-quarter of patients
polled said they waited two hours or more.

Harris has heard, as have all nurses, stories about increasing physical violence against emergency-room nurses,* but she has not experienced it first-hand. Triage nurses are nonetheless equipped with emergency buzzers that will bring immediate help.

Like all nursing specialties, triage attracts nurses with particular skills. Harris not only has done the job for a long time, but is now responsible for hiring others. The public can be very demanding, so a particular demeanour is required on the front line of Emergency. Critical skills and problem-solving skills are the most important traits, but the triage nurse also needs to be "empathetic, non-judgmental, and thick-skinned," she says.

While non-urgent cases have made up the majority of patients for the thirty years Harris has worked in Emergency, they are becoming more problematic today, for a couple of reasons. First, because the minority of cases that are truly emergencies are far more acute. Second, because there are fewer nurses as a result of a combination of cutbacks and shortages. That means the lulls that used to allow nurses and physicians to clear up the backlog of non-urgent cases simply don't happen anymore.

A mid-size hospital like St. John's General sees about 40,000 patients a year. There are eleven exam rooms in Emergency (soon to be twenty-four). There are usually six or seven nurses. Twenty patients in the waiting room is not uncommon, especially in the evening. (Emergency tends to have its busy time from 4:00 P.M. to 2:00 A.M.) From a management perspective—a role Harris has stepped into recently—the most difficult part of emergency nursing is its unpredictability.

The veterans have learned some of the signs, Harris says. On clear, sunny days, there will be an influx of patients, particularly older ones, "who have things they just want looked at but that are not emergencies." Heavy fog and rain translates into motor-vehicle accidents. The first heavy snow of the season, a rash of back

---

* A 1999 study found that 60 per cent of ER nurses had been physically assaulted in the past year, and more than half of them said that fear of violence impairs their ability to provide quality care.

injuries and severed fingers from snowblowers. Warm summer nights mean alcohol poisoning and stabbings, and car crashes brought about by impaired driving.

While statistically about 100 patients a day visit the General's emergency department, the flow of patients and the severity of their conditions can vary wildly from one hour to the next. Some days all the patients will flood in over a four-hour period; on other days, there will be a steady trickle over twenty-four hours. "You can have a whole morning of stubbed toes, and get into a lazy mode, then all of a sudden there are a couple of major traumas, coupled with a large influx of patients. That's when we say: 'Oh-oh, the bus has pulled up,'" Harris says. What the triage nurse likes, above all, is a rhythm, having patients arrive in a steady flow rather than in peaks and valleys.

Harris believes that the overcrowding problem is chronic and systemic, and that it will remain until those who formulate health policies and priorities decide to resolve emergency-room backlogs once and for all. She believes politicians want to have it both ways: they want to cut back on costs but shield the public from the reality for fear of a backlash. That creates artificial expectations. "Everybody thinks that Emergency is the place to go for all your aches and pains, and no one has taught them otherwise. We should promote the reality of the emergency room a lot more. People need to know that, with limited resources, the wait will be long for a minor problem. Some cases will take six hours, there's no doubt about it. But no one is being denied emergency treatment. These are patients who can be seen elsewhere and, if they knew the reality, maybe they would go elsewhere," Harris says.

Patients often do not realize that Emergency was one of the areas of health care hit first and hardest when shortages began to happen. In secondary centres like St. John's General, recruitment is a constant preoccupation, filling shifts from one day to the next a constant worry. "There's a nursing crisis out there that impacts us every day, and it's only going to get worse," Harris says. When full-time staff is hard to come by, having part-timers on call—

something necessary to deal with the unpredictability of ER—is all the more difficult. So full-time nurses end up doing a lot of overtime, and burning out.

For Harris, relief will come only when the problem of non-urgent patients is addressed squarely and firmly. She warns grimly that "education is something that's really lacking. The public needs to learn the proper use of Emergency. If they don't, they're going to be faced with a situation where Emergency is not available to them when they really do have a serious problem."

An Open Wound—Anthony Arsenault

"What is the most important trait of a burn nurse?" asks Anthony Arsenault, repeating the question. "Definitely, a strong stomach. There is no question the job can be grotesque, the work disgusting. The odour from the mouth, or from the fluid bubbling out of the nose of a patient can be vile. When you remove a dressing, a wave of smell hits you that is worse than anything you can imagine. But, honest to God, I can't imagine doing anything else."

Arsenault is a nurse at the Ross Tilley Burn Unit of the Sunnybrook and Women's College Health Sciences Centre, one of the most demanding and specialized jobs in nursing today. Severe burn victims—those who have had thousands of volts of electricity course through their body, those who are doused in corrosive chemicals, scalded by high-pressure steam, or seared by flames—are probably the sickest of the sick. That is because skin, the body's largest organ, is a person's primary defence against infection. Burn victims cannot regulate their temperature, maintain their bodily fluids, keep their blood pressure stable, or fight off even the most mundane virus or bacteria. They are, quite literally, an open wound.

Despite the visual and olfactory demands, Arsenault loves the challenge of wound management and understands the process of healing. Seemingly simple tasks, such as changing dressings, can mean the difference between life and death for patients. "The beauty of dressing duty is that it looks like a menial job, but it is really specialized work. Knowing how to read a wound is an art. It's not looking at a monitor or reading a number, it's being attuned to subtle changes in the body. And it's really rewarding because I use my knowledge to care for people."

When burn victims come to the hospital, they go directly to the hydrotherapy room, or the tub room. There was a time when they were plunged into a tub of water, but today they are laid on a stainless-steel stretcher and washed continually with a series of hoses. Doctors will install an intravenous line, a central line (usually in the groin), an internal monitor for arterial pressure, and a catheter; they may also intubate (insert a tube into an organ), or chemically paralyse the patient or induce a coma. Nurses are responsible for monitoring vital signs, doing continual assessment, and ensuring there is an adequate supply of fluids and blood products on hand. (Severe burn victims may get up to 300 units of blood.) It is messy work because fluids pour out of every part of the patient's body. It is also oppressively hot because the room is heated to body temperature, since patients are not able to regulate their temperature, and medical personnel are covered head to toe to minimize the risk of infection.

A nurse might spend three hours straight in the tub room, but it is afterwards that the real work begins. "When you're in the tub room, you know the family is just outside the door, filled with fear and terror, and you're going to have to deal with them soon," Arsenault says. Once the patient is stabilized, debridement (the removal of dead skin) begins, then wounds are treated with anti-microbal fluid and wrapped with special gauze. There may be several rounds of surgery, including amputations. Then the long process of healing begins.

Patients are so damaged and so volatile that they get virtually one-on-one care. The nurse will monitor and assess regularly, on the lookout for the slightest sign of infection. The fourteen beds at Ross Tilley are each in an isolation room. Each shift, one nurse will be assigned to dressing duty. Others are responsible for pain management and other tasks, and lot of time is spent with families.

"I've seen hundreds of these cases and I still can't imagine the sense of horror, the feeling of hopelessness that's always on the mind of the spouse, mother, or family member. They're out of their minds with grief and fear. I address it by getting them involved. If a wife is sobbing at the bedside, I say: 'Do you want to give me a hand? Do you want to wipe his face?' They love it. They feel they are contributing to care," Arsenault says.

Burn patients will spend up to a year in the unit, from the initial trauma through to rehabilitation, so nurses get to know them and their families intimately. For the first month or two, victims will be treated with heavy doses of narcotics, kept virtually in a coma. The hardest part of nursing is when the patient emerges from this period. Newly conscious, he or she is often in extreme pain, in addition to dealing with some major psychological issues. "It's an intense period in the nurse–patient relationship. It's also the key part of the healing process," Arsenault says.

During this make-it-or-break-it period, the nurse focuses on pain management, trying to make the pain bearable while still allowing patients to think clearly and have input into their treatment. "At this point, the human stuff is way more important to me than the medical stuff. When you see this person in front of you who is absolutely terrified and you know you can help, that's what caring is all about. That's the essence of nursing," he explains.

Because of the gravity of the injuries and the raw feelings the healing process unleashes in patients, many nurses get quite emotionally involved. "I get so moved by the journey that I'm reduced to tears sometimes—we all are. Just seeing a patient standing in a doorway all alone after so many months of suffering just floors me. There are days I say: 'Oh my God. These people are walking miracles.'"

For burn nurses, seeing the daily litany of horrific injuries is maddening because the vast majority occur in preventable accidents: throwing gasoline on the barbecue, touching an electric wire with a metal ladder, taking a shortcut around safety procedures when working with chemicals. It is not fire or electricity that kills, but carelessness. Handymen and hydro workers are often at risk, but the nurse has never seen a firefighter pass through the burn unit. The most difficult cases to deal with on a personal basis, however, are the elderly (there are no pediatric cases at Ross Tilley). Most seniors suffer injuries from scalding, usually dropping pots of hot water or caught in a too-hot shower because of mobility problems.

Arsenault says one of the haunting aspects of his job is caring for patients who are perfectly lucid, but who are burned so severely that they have essentially lost the ability to feel. "I can be sitting there with an old guy and he's just chatting away, telling funny stories, and looking at his wounds, I just know he will be dead in two days. It breaks my heart."

Because of medical advances, most burn patients who do not die on site will survive. But there are still a lot of deaths. Surprisingly, Arsenault finds that is not a difficult part of his work. Far more troubling than those quick deaths are the patients who worked hard for months at recovery only to be felled by a virus or bacteria that most healthy people could fight off. Frustratingly, despite all the precautions, infection remains the number one killer of burn victims.

Like many nurses today, Arsenault is a part-time employee who works full-time hours, meaning he gets no benefits and no pension plan. He has also experienced the upheaval of a hospital merger. When Wellesley Hospital was gobbled up by the giant Sunnybrook as part of Ontario's "restructuring," the renowned burn centre moved. Physically, the facilities are much improved, brand new and state of the art. But while nurses and doctors moved to the new site with the unit, the specialized health-care aides did not, because of union issues. "We all work together as a team, and we had to leave an invaluable part of that team behind with the merger. On paper, it looks fine, but the people who dream up these things never bother with the important details that make a difference in patient care," Arsenault observes.

He is quick to add, however, that he could not imagine a better job, because it's one of the only areas in nursing today where you still build bonds, lasting bonds. "Nurses get to know patients and their families very well over several months, and, when they leave, walking on their own, you really know you have made a difference to a lot of lives."

Searching for Hope—Wendy Morrison

University of British Columbia Hospital is home to the largest multiple sclerosis (MS) clinic in the world. More than 4,000 patients flock there because the facility is at the cutting edge in the search for treatments—and ultimately a cure—for the devastating neurological disease.

"A decade ago, a physician would sit down with a newly diagnosed patient and say: 'You have multiple sclerosis. There's nothing we can do. Come back when you need a wheelchair.' Since then, there have been a number of advances, so we treat early and treat aggressively," says Wendy Morrison, a nurse and research coordinator for MS clinical research. Sitting in a tiny office overflowing with paper, poring over data late into the evening, she looks more like an overwhelmed graduate student than someone stretching the boundaries of nursing. But Morrison is actually a key partner on a team that includes five neurology nurses and six neurologists who are probing the effectiveness of new drugs and their impact on the quality of life of people with MS. This backroom work has repercussions around the world.

Morrison toils in relative anonymity, but the dramatic advances in the MS field have been closely tied to her career as a researcher. Her first research project involved Betaseron (also known as interferon beta-1b), the first-ever drug that slowed progression of the disease. "That was really exciting: Just imagine how it felt to be able to offer people treatment for a disease for the first time." But the research showed that the drug worked with only a very select group (about 30 per cent), and it fell largely to nurses to tell the other 70 per cent of sufferers why it would not help them.

After initial success came a "period where everything we tried failed miserably. That really gets you down because people are counting on you," Morrison says. "But you keep going because you know this work will ultimately make a big difference to a lot of people."

MS is a neurological disease with a genetic component, but its progression is probably influenced by environmental and medical factors. The gene that carries MS has not yet been identified, nor have the triggers. (One theory is that the virus herpes 6 may spur the disease in people who are predisposed.)* An autoimmune disease, it affects more than twice as many women as men. Clinic patients range in age from 19 to 65, but most start to suffer symptoms at mid-life, when they have careers and families. MS is not fatal generally, but is the equivalent of smoking a pack of cigarettes a day in terms of reducing life expectancy. (People with MS used to die of bladder problems related to nervous-system breakdown, but treatment of symptoms has improved dramatically.) It also effects mobility, and therefore lifestyle.

MS affects the myelin (a protective sheath of proteins) on nerve fibres. Today, there are three different interferon-based treatments† that aim to slow the breakdown of myelin. Copaxone, a newer non-interferon treatment, alters the way the immune system works in the brain. The treatments are expensive, ranging from $11,800 to $22,000 annually. Most patients do not pay the full cost, but governments are becoming increasingly reluctant to subsidize, which has prompted many nurses to become advocates for their patients. Morrison, for example, is on the board of directors of the MS Society of British Columbia. Patients who participate in drug trials, of course, pay nothing.

Drug trials are long, complicated affairs that involve a lot of paperwork, take a lot of time, raise all kinds of ethical issues, and

---

* The risk of contracting MS is about 1 in 1,000 among people of Eastern European descent. If you have a sibling with MS, your risk rises to about 1 in 20.
† Rebif, Avanex, and Betaseron.

depend on a solid team of investigators. MS studies can last three years or longer. Paradoxically, much of the research focuses on people who are well; because nerve damage cannot be repaired, efforts have concentrated on protecting myelin. But drugs like interferon have nasty side effects, and it is not always easy to convince healthy people to take them in the hope their health will be maintained over the long term.

Morrison says this reality is one of the reasons nurses play such a prominent role in research. "Simply put, what nurses do best is recruit people and keep them coming back. When trials last for years and, from the point of view of patients, seem to do diddly-squat—except maybe make them sick—that's invaluable. A lot of studies would die if we didn't have nurses so involved."

Nurses create loyalty because they offer patients more than drugs and a battery of follow-up tests. As nurses do their research, they provide counselling and education that patients cannot get anywhere else. "We do surveys, and the patients say the best part of research is having regular contact with someone who is knowledgeable about their condition," Morrison says. "Patients with a chronic disease need to vent. Generally, they don't want to complain to a spouse or friends, they want to stay upbeat in their daily lives. And the best thing about complaining to a nurse is that we can often deal with complaints in a useful way; we can offer not only sympathy, but solutions." Many of those complaints, or the observations nurses make while doing drug studies, serve as the basis for other research.

The independent nursing research tends to focus on patients rather than on the biology of the disease. For example, clinic staff have always wondered why some people cope very well with a diagnosis while others fall apart, so nurses are trying to discover the factors that influence the coping mechanisms. They also do research on the link between progression of the disease and clinical depression.

Morrison loves her work, but a constant frustration is that nurses don't tend to get much credit for research. While she stresses that her colleagues at the University of British Columbia Hospital are very professional ("They tend to give credit where it's due"), speaking more generally the nurse says that the core of research—the daily collection of data, the hand-holding of clients to ensure compliance, the crunching of numbers, and the early waving of flags when there are problems—is the responsibility of the nurses, not the physicians who write the final reports.

While Morrison is one of the most highly specialized nurses in the country, the monetary rewards for such expertise are skimpy. She earns about $10,000 a year less as a researcher than what she earned as a neurology nurse in a hospital. She also has no job security. For the past dozen years, she has had a series of six-month contracts, and their renewal is entirely grant-dependent. The clinic gets only a fraction of its budget from the hospital; most funding comes from research grants from drug companies.

In Morrison's experience, private enterprise, where efficiency and results are paramount, is far more supportive of nursing practice than the public sector. "The pharmaceutical industry realizes the value of nurses. They demand a nursing coordinator on all projects, and the involvement of nurses. They know that, otherwise, they won't be able to recruit and retain patients." The other, unspoken role of the nursing coordinator is to keep the principal investigator honest, to ensure that corners are not cut and data not falsified. (The huge scandals in the United States, and to a lesser extent in Canada, in recent years over doctored data more often than not involved projects that did not have a nursing component.)

Morrison has repeatedly been offered jobs in the pharmaceutical industry—at much higher pay, she adds with a sigh—but has turned them down because she does not want to lose direct patient contact. She found the transition from high-octane neurological intensive care to more mellow neurological research to be difficult enough. She doesn't want to move entirely away from hands-on nursing.

"In neuroscience, we're in the business of hope. We can't cure people, all we can do is help them find hope to carry on in a different way. I don't want to just push paper around. I want to be there, on the ground, in the clinic, squeezing out a little bit more hope every day."

The Journey of Care — Colleen Harris

When the media write about disease, the focus is often on finding a cure. But one would be hard-pressed to identify even one major illness (aside from infectious diseases for which vaccines have been developed) that has been cured. Rather, medical advances for diseases with a genetic component often involve the control of symptoms, or the delay of their onset. Illnesses that were once debilitating or fatal have become manageable and chronic. In other words, the search for cures, to which nurses such as Wendy Morrison contribute enormously, has resulted in an exponential growth in the need for care.

The multiple sclerosis (MS) clinic at Foothills Health Centre in Calgary, for example, had a single nurse a decade ago. Today, it has five. Colleen Harris, a nurse-practitioner, is part of the team. "I do a lot of the work neurologists used to do. This way patients get way more access to the specialty care they need," she says.

In MS, neurological breakdown allows immune cells to penetrate the brain, destroying nerves and scrambling signals. The use of magnetic resonance imaging (MRI) technology to catch this phenomenon early has allowed early diagnosis. Unfortunately, the only effective treatments that exist today are for people in the early stages of the disease. "The focus of our practice has changed completely in a very short time. We have gone from focusing on disability, on preparing people for inevitable disability, to seeing people in early stages and putting them on medication to prevent disability. I've been blessed to see dramatic change and, because of it, I can barely imagine a field of work that is more rewarding for a nurse right now," Harris says.

Her principal task is designing treatment plans for the newcomers to the ranks of MS. When new drugs are approved, when new research is published about advances in the field, her role is to interpret it for the patients, and incorporate it in their treatment. Working on salary, rather than fee-for-service, Harris offers thorough clinic assessment visits, usually taking ninety minutes. She does a physical and neurological examination, with particular emphasis on the movement impairments caused by the disease. She does a detailed review of physical and neurological changes since the previous visit, probes the effects and side effects of medication, and modifies the treatment plan as needed. The nurse then dictates letters to the patient's neurologist and family physician, to update them on the treatment plan. (In a field such as MS, knowledge has become so specialized and advances so rapid that family practitioners now routinely turn to specialized nurses for advice and guidance.)

The only things Harris cannot do that a doctor can are make an initial diagnosis and directly prescribe drugs, but "this is not a significant barrier at all," she says. The nurse can order tests, interpret findings, and make referrals to other specialists. She is also responsible for maintenance of interstitial pump and pack technology, an implant that helps deliver drugs directly to a patient's system on a regulated basis (instead of requiring them to inject).

For three days a week, Harris has face-to-face clinic appointments. On the other two days, she is responsible for triage duties in the community, determining, for example, if a patient with MS requires home care. And much of her time is spent dealing with crises, whether physical, social, or a combination of the two. For example, a patient with an acute exacerbation of MS symptoms will usually be rushed into treatment with steroids. But it is the emotional issues that are more common and harder to deal with. "A typical crisis call is a patient who calls and says 'My husband has left, he can't take it anymore.' It's not unusual for there to be talk of suicide.* When those calls came, I used to get in the car and go over there, but union guidelines now prevent us from doing

---

* The suicide rate among people with MS is seven times that of the general population.

that. Now I have to coordinate the help. I will involve the social worker, the home-care nurse, maybe an MS Society volunteer. We do what we have to, to help," Harris says.

With diseases like MS that hit in the prime of life, and often without warning, there is a lot of anger, and people often lash out at their caregiver. Part of the nurse's role is to deal with those emotions. Half as many men get MS, but they often suffer far greater damage, and don't cope as well as women. "Maybe it's the stigma," Harris hypothesizes. Regardless of people's emotions, the benefit of a clinic is that it is always there when people need to deal with issues over the many years they will have the chronic disease.

An experienced intensive-care neurology nurse, Harris worked several years in major Los Angeles hospitals. "In the United States, they offer specialized nurses the moon, and they deliver," she says. The job was great, the educational opportunities wonderful, and the pay superb, but Harris had trouble working in a system that does not guarantee access to care to everyone, as Canada does. "After a while, you realize what U.S. health is all about. It's about making money. It's not about caring for everyone who needs help," she points out.

The clinic clientele in Calgary features everyone from corporate executives to recipients of social assistance. While they all get equal care, Harris worries about the fact that access is getting more difficult. MS is not a fatal disease, so patients rarely need to be hospitalized. But, in the later stages of the disease, when motor functions break down, patients do need help. When Harris started at the clinic, there came a point at which patients were admitted to long-term-care facilities. That doesn't happen anymore. And while her patients tend to have a better quality of life with home care, she gets angry when the wait for approval stretches into months or when the hours allocated for care are clearly inadequate. Similarly, access to rehabilitation or to the services of an occupational therapist is getting increasingly difficult to guarantee in an era of cutbacks.

"MS is a chronic disease, but it can be managed. If you design a good treatment plan and the services are available, you can keep people working and in the community, and keep them healthier a lot longer. But, often, the way services are cut, or limited, is quite short-sighted. If you limit rehab now, you are going to pay for that down the road," Harris advises.

The nurse-practitioner feels that dealing with chronic illness is one of the great challenges for the Canadian health system. Designed principally to treat, then discharge patients, the system has to adapt to the reality that an increasing number of patients—and probably the majority in the near future—will need, not quick hits, but continual treatment for many, many years.

"I follow them through the journey, I see them for a lifetime. It's the kind of nursing a lot of us dream of doing," Harris says. "I'm not like a typical hospital nurse; I'm not down. My morale is really good. This is a good place to be in nursing today. And it will be an even better place tomorrow."

Managing Loss — Cheryl Magnusson

There are more than eighty types of autoimmune diseases. What they have in common is that the symptoms—fatigue and debilitating pain—are not outwardly visible. The vast majority of sufferers are also women, young women who look healthy but have to deal with enormous psychological and financial repercussions. Their caregivers tend to be women too—nurses.

Cheryl Magnusson is a rheumatology nurse at the Mary Pack Arthritis Centre in Vancouver, Canada's only free-standing arthritis centre.* She deals principally with the two best-known autoimmune disorders, rheumatoid arthritis† and lupus. There is no cure for either, but there are various treatments, most of which suppress the immune system or try to control pain.

"Our patients take a lot of powerful drugs with potentially

---

* Operated independently by the Arthritis Society of Canada until 1997, the centre is now administered by Vancouver Hospital.
† Rheumatoid arthritis is not the same as osteoarthritis, a degenerative joint disease common in the elderly.

dangerous side effects," explains Magnusson. In fact, treatments can resemble chemotherapy, though patients will also get injections of corticosteroids and gold.* Most nurses in the clinic will oversee these treatments and do drug monitoring. They will see fifty to sixty patients daily and take many more phone calls from people suffering various side effects.

Magnusson will pitch in occasionally, but her principal role is to deal with everything that cannot be treated with drugs, everything else that flows from having a chronic disease that leaves you in constant pain and perpetually exhausted. "The counselling I do centres on loss. When you develop arthritis or other autoimmune diseases, you lose a lot of things: You can lose your job, your functional abilities; above all, you lose the person you thought you would be the rest of your life."

She teaches pain management and sleep management. (There are a lot of sleep disturbances brought on by joint pain and the side effects of drugs.) Similarly, diet and nutrition play a key role in coping with the disease. A woman with arthritis who is overweight will put undue stress on her joints; a woman with lupus who eats poorly can exacerbate renal damage. A man in the early stages of ankylosing spondylitis† can worsen spinal damage if he has a poorly designed work station.

Many people are diagnosed with autoimmune disorders in their thirties and forties, when they have families and careers, and the changes can be shocking. "I find myself doing lots of counselling on body image. Women who have always felt good about themselves can lose their hair, or end up with deformities; the medications can alter their appearance, or interfere with their ability to conceive," says Magnusson. "These are big issues but they don't really get dealt with in the traditional medical model."

---

* Gold salts in injectable form are sometimes used in the treatment of rheumatoid arthritis.
† Ankylosing spondylitis, also known as "bamboo spine," is a condition in which the spinal vertebrae fuse together, causing debilitating stiffness. It primarily affects men under the age of 30.

She can, by no means, do all of this alone. The nurse will see two to six patients daily, often for lengthy sessions, and at various hours. Because many patients do not want any further disruptions in their work or family lives, they will make appointments in the evening or early in the morning, and Magnusson allows them this flexibility. She will also make referrals to other specialists in the centre and in the community, such as dieticians, physiotherapists, nephrologists, psychologists, and social workers. "These patients have complex cases that include all kinds of physical, psychological, and financial issues. So, a large part of my work is coordinating communications between the disciplines. The communication role falls naturally on nurses," Magnusson says. Another increasingly important aspect of that role is doing public speaking about arthritis, both to other nurses and to members of the general public.*

The approach the clinic takes is goal-setting, allowing patients to set realistic targets for the management of their disease. When they are stable, they are often discharged from the program, but because they will be living with the condition the rest of their lives, the clinic is always open to them. This lack of finality or resolution does not frustrate Magnusson at all; on the contrary, she likes being viewed as a long-term resource.

"I left acute care because it was so frustrating that I was burning out. We would discharge patients and see them again in two months in worse condition. We dealt with acuity, with the crisis, but there was no disease management. It was depressing to see all these people on a treadmill when you knew they could be helped a lot more another way."

She sees the specialized clinic as an ideal approach to treating people with chronic disease, and a wonderful setting for the practice of nursing. A clinic allows patients to have control over their treatment, and it allows nurses to practise holistically. "With diseases like lupus, there's scientific evidence that, if people feel

* Some clinic employees are paid directly by the Arthritis Society, but Magnusson is not.

more in control, they have less disease activity, so these strategies really work," Magnusson says.

Like many nurses today, she is pursuing higher education while working. Magnusson's master's thesis focuses on how people with rheumatoid arthritis make health-care choices. She is finding that, in the traditional health-care model, many patients feel excluded and, as a result, have a tendency to let the disease degenerate before seeking care. That way, they are far more likely to end up in Emergency and cost the system a lot more money than ongoing clinic visits do. Getting people involved is particularly important and cost-effective with diseases like lupus, where patients often walk a fine line between managing well and needing hospitalization.

"It's easy to demonstrate what an emergency-room nurse does. It's a lot more difficult to demonstrate to people exactly what we do in a clinic to keep patients healthy and out of hospital. There isn't enough recognition of how important it is to keep patients informed and in control, and how that pays dividends. Nurses have the knowledge base about disease and medication, and we know how other health professionals can contribute to the well-being of the individual. When we're given an ability to use those skills, it can have a real impact," Magnusson argues.

There is a lot of pressure on nurses today to do research, pressure both from employers and in academia. While that may bring welcome attention to the profession, it is not always in the best interest of patients, who see caring take a back seat to prodding and poking. Magnusson's job is a throwback to the days when the principal role of the nurse—because there were so few treatments and cures—was prevention and minimizing the impact of illnesses on patients and their families. "What I like about this type of nursing is [that] the frame of reference is not the disease, it's the person. I'm helping people with health management, and that's something that's really lacking in our system today."

No Ifs, Ands, or Butts—Carol McDonald

Carol McDonald is polite to a fault and speaks in a quiet voice. Sitting in a modest cubicle in a west-end Ottawa office building, surrounded by posters and paper, she hardly looks like a threat. But for the past decade, day in and day out, McDonald has been staring down Canada's most prolific killer and battling a unrepentant poisoner—and she's winning.

McDonald is a nurse with the Region of Ottawa–Carleton Public Health Unit, a veteran of its tobacco information division. With missionary zeal, she sets out each day to get smokers to quit and to expand the legal protections for non-smokers. She does so effectively but, like many nurses, invisibly. "As usual, in public health, nurses do a lot of work in the background, behind the scenes. But that doesn't matter. What matters is that it works, that we make a difference in people's lives," McDonald says.

The Ottawa region has fewer smokers than almost anywhere else in the country: 22 per cent of adults smoke daily, and twice as many have never smoked; 31 per cent are former smokers. Since McDonald started her work, the number of smokers in the area has fallen by 10 per cent. (In most of the rest of the country, after a steady twenty-five-year decline, rates are on the increase again, particularly among teenagers.) "That's gratifying, but one in five still smokes, and they have a 50 per cent chance of dying of smoking-related illnesses. That's such a waste," McDonald says.

Ontario's Chief Medical Officer of Health warned, in a 1997 report, that tobacco use costs the provincial economy $10 million and kills thirty-three people daily.* He concluded that, unless efforts are redoubled, "we are in danger of losing the war against tobacco."

McDonald has approached her public-health duties like a military tactician, drafting elaborate plans, studying her enemy's every move, and continually adjusting the strategy. In 1991, after provincial-government funds were made available for anti-tobacco campaigns,

---

* Worldwide more than 10,000 people die daily from the effects of tobacco.

the nurse, along with a physician, wrote what they called a "comprehensive plan of attack," and they were awarded the biggest grant. The strategy was four-pronged: reduce the number of adult smokers; prevent young people from smoking; protect the environment for non-smokers; and promote smoking cessation.

Within each of these categories, there have been a number of initiatives over the years. The public-health department set up a Tobacco Information Line that is staffed by nurses. People can call for the latest medical information, for statistical data about smoking, and for referrals to community programs to help them quit. The unit subsidizes smoking-cessation programs, so they can be offered free of charge. It also promotes legislative change, from advocating municipal bylaws to make public spaces and workplaces smoke-free to calling for the federal government to increase taxes on tobacco products. And a team of public-health nurses dedicates itself exclusively to educating teens, in the hope that they will prevent them from smoking.* The area has become so specialized that one nurse works full-time with pregnant teens, another with elementary-school children, and yet another on relapse prevention.†

McDonald also spends an increasingly large part of her time on social marketing, creating campaigns designed to change deeply rooted notions that smoking is cool, and an issue of personal choice rather than one of public health. Part of that job is running an annual poster contest.

She also does a lot of education work, such as teaching physicians and nurses in other settings how they can successfully help people to quit smoking. "We used to just say: 'Don't smoke.' Obviously, that didn't work. We realize now there are all kinds of societal and environmental factors that influence smoking, and that we have to attack the problem on many fronts at the same time if we're going to be successful," McDonald suggests.

She marvels at how much knowledge has changed in the time

* More than 50 per cent of children try smoking by age 12; of those who have not smoked before the age of 19, only a tiny fraction ever take up the habit.
† The average smoker takes six tries before quitting successfully.

she has been involved in the field, but the chronic indifference about the ravages of smoking has made her more determined over the years. "I've been involved with smokers my entire career, since graduation in 1966. One of my first jobs was suctioning COPDers [those suffering from chronic obstructive pulmonary disorder]. I had at least one patient a week who needed surgery for lung disease," McDonald says. She went from Hôtel-Dieu in Kingston to St. Mary's Hospital in Montreal, to the Ottawa Heart Institute. She spent fourteen years at the last organization, working in preadmission, surgery, and post-op, much of her time spent teaching heart patients and their families about the dangers of smoking.

"I've seen so much pain related to smoking, it's unbelievable. All that time in hospital, seeing the hearts and lungs and lives that were destroyed by tobacco, prepared me for this job doing prevention," McDonald says. "I left the Heart Institute with tobacco stamped on my soul as the number one problem in society."

Today, the bulk of McDonald's job is grass-roots advocacy. She sits on the board of directors of the Lung Association and, in a non-official capacity, is a member of the Ottawa–Carleton Council on Smoking and Health, a group that succeeded in getting the local airport to go smoke-free. As a public-health nurse, McDonald focuses much of her energy on protecting the 80 per cent of non-smokers from the dangers and bother of second-hand smoke. This is often tedious, plodding work. She has been working for more than six years to make one subsidized housing project for seniors smoke-free, not only to help those individuals, but in the hope it will set a small precedent. Similarly, she has allied prisoners and staff at a small correctional facility in a bid to make it smoke-free. And the nurse spends countless hours trying to convince municipal councillors of the wisdom of implementing anti-smoking bylaws.

McDonald operates in this manner because she is convinced public-health initiatives are most powerful at the local level. "To quote Victor Crawford:* 'Tobacco companies fear political action

* A long-time lawyer for U.S. tobacco companies, he died of lung cancer.

at the local level the most because it's there that they have the least influence,'" she says.

The nurse is openly disdainful of the reluctance of the provincial and federal governments to make a concerted effort against tobacco. The cut in federal and provincial tobacco taxes (a policy aimed at reducing smuggling) infuriated her, and the refusal to treat tobacco as a dangerous substance disgusts her. "Every person who uses this product has a 50 per cent chance of dying of smoking-related illness. We do not accept that in any other additive, or any other consumer product. In this country, they don't regulate tobacco as much as they do orange juice," McDonald says, placing the blame squarely on politicians who are influenced more by big-money lobbying by tobacco companies than by a concern for public health.

McDonald studies the methods of the tobacco industry carefully, and dreams of the day when the public-health teams will be able to fight back with equal arms, and similar budgets. She wonders why governments allow themselves to continue misspending on treatment of lung and heart disease instead of investing in prevention. For example, the public-health nurse has been lobbying for government to subsidize new pharmacotherapies for smokers who want to quit, and to make smoking-cessation courses available free of charge. (Ottawa is the exception in this regard.) "You can get open-heart surgery at no charge in this country, but you have to pay for the [nicotine] patch. How does that make any sense? You can buy a lot of patches, and you can prevent a lot of heart disease, for the cost of one surgery." McDonald, an inveterate letter writer, has, of course, demanded answers to these questions. The person responsible for the Ontario drug-benefits plan once told her that the plan initially paid for Nicorette gum, but there was abuse, so smoking-cessation methods are no longer subsidized.

McDonald certainly has not given up on that issue, but realizes that her work is cumulative and that she will see real results only in the long term. In the meantime, she takes great joy in the little victories; the former smoker who calls the Tobacco Information Line to say, "thanks," the restaurant that declares itself smoke-free, the teenager who wins the latest anti-smoking-poster contest. McDonald even speaks proudly of her father who, at age 78, finally quit smoking. "It was hard to see my dad smoking, but he was stubborn and didn't want my help. I didn't want the tobacco industry interfering with my relationship with my dad, so I didn't push it. But others talked to him, and he quit, and his health has improved."

To McDonald, that the anti-smoking message could get through even to her father shows that people are listening, and that her work is all worthwhile. "I'm not here to cause smokers any hardship, I'm here to support non-smokers. And I think some day people are going to look back and wonder why there weren't a lot more public-health nurses like me around a lot sooner."

Mending Your Business—Lynda Kushnir Pekrul

In a typical week, more than 500,000 Canadians, or 6 per cent of the workforce, are off the job with a variety of illnesses. Sick days cost the economy and employers billions of dollars annually in paid leave and lost productivity. But if it is a given that healthy employees are more productive and profitable, what are businesses doing to promote wellness? The answer, unfortunately, is: not very much.

One exception is the insurance industry, which aggressively promotes healthy living among its employees. It does so by building in-house clinics and staffing them with occupational-health nurses.

Canada Life is typical. Its main office tower in Regina's business district features a resplendent health centre that consists of a clinic, a quiet room, a health library, and an ergonomics room. It employs a medical director who is a physician (but who does not see patients) and two full-time nurses. "A lot of what insurers do is ultimately influenced by public-health issues, so they give this a lot of thought. The fact that companies recognize this service as essential should tell us something about its value," says Lynda Kushnir Pekrul, one of the centre's nurses.*

* She has since started working at Health Canada in health promotion for aboriginals.

With 1,200 employees, Canada Life is a microcosm of the outside world, so the parade of aches and pains that passes through the clinic is varied. People come in for over-the-counter medication, to change dressings, to have their blood pressure checked, for diabetic monitoring, or for relief from migraines. But treating illnesses that arise in the workplace is just a pretext for doing longer-term prevention work.

"An employee will say: 'I have a headache and would like a couple of Tylenol.' Well, they probably have Tylenol in their desk and what they really want to do is talk about what's really bothering them," Kushnir Pekrul says. That larger issue could be the stress of caring for an elderly parent, the inability to conceive, or concern over weight gain, all issues that could have a significant impact on job performance if they are not dealt with promptly.

Kushnir Pekrul knows that her role is helping people come to grips with issues and then navigate through the health-care system. She understands that there is really no other place in that system where people can go for advice. Family physicians used to serve in that role, but they rarely take more than a few minutes per patient and are not always accessible when a question pops up, whereas, in the workplace, any employee can drop into the clinic at lunch or during a coffee break.

"They might make a doctor's appointment because of a sore stomach; the physician will diagnose something, then say: 'Take this pill.' So much has happened, they don't have any questions. But, later, when it's time to take the pill, they have all kinds of questions. We sit down with the patients and help them understand," Kushnir Pekrul says. "As the health-care system has been shut down and people get shuffled around, they are increasingly looking for this kind of clinic. We offer a personal touch, and we fill in a lot of the blanks."

As someone with a background in the intensive care unit (ICU) and cardiology, Kushnir Pekrul feels this is a different kind of nursing, and a different kind of satisfaction as a nurse. There aren't the highs and lows of ICU. The success stories are wrapped up in slowly unfolding life events. It's much longer-term work than in a hospital. But the clinic offers a chance to do what many nurses long to do—get to know their patients, and share in their little triumphs: the couple who work through infertility; the guy who kicks the three-pack-a-day habit; the woman who finds the comfortable exercise and nutrition program that has long evaded her. The downside is that, when you know clients well, the inevitable life crises that arise—miscarriages, death in the family, disabilities from traffic accidents, a cancer diagnosis—affect a nurse more deeply.

What the clinic demonstrates is that, when given the resources to do so, many people will take greater interest in and responsibility for their good health. A company like Canada Life has a workforce that is healthy and is looking for wellness advice, not treatment for illness. That, too, is hard to come by in the beleaguered public-health system. So the clinic offers advice on nutrition, fitness, smoking cessation, and stress management, both one on one and in group sessions. The clinic is also the link to a more formal employee-assistance program, where people can get professional counselling for issues such as alcoholism, drug abuse, relationship problems, and sexual dysfunction.

In a work environment where a lot of people are doing repetitive tasks such as data entry and data analysis—most of it sitting at a desk, staring at a computer screen—there is a lot of emphasis on avoiding repetitive strain injury (RSI), a scourge of the modern office. The nurse teaches RSI prevention, and a massage therapist comes into the clinic four days a week. (Each employee is allowed up to $350 annually in therapeutic massage.)

The company also invests heavily in ergonomics. The occupational-health nurse who works with Kushnir Pekrul does individual analyses of each work station to ensure that it is comfortable, in order to reduce the likelihood of RSI, back problems, and eye strain. She even has a budget to purchase all sorts of gadgets to adapt the already-modern furniture and accessories. Because the environment affects productivity, it's a good investment; avoiding problems now is easier than trying to treat injuries later.

Aside from working with patients, Kushnir Pekrul carries out a number of administrative functions related to her background as an occupational-health nurse. For example, she deals with Workers' Compensation Board claims and supervises the company's disability-leave program. (Insurance companies employ a lot of nurses on the policy side to verify that claims are medically legitimate, but Kushnir Pekrul works on the employee side, as an advocate.) At Canada Life, employees obviously have good disability insurance. But how the company distinguishes itself is in the way it adapts to a worker's return—whether after a car accident or treatment for a heart condition or other chronic disability. Kushnir Pekrul will reconfigure the workplace to the needs of those workers, and can even establish flexible hours that take into consideration tiredness or a physiotherapy regime. "Our goal is to get people back to work, because we know a job can play a big part in building self-esteem and in healing," she explains.

The nurse also ensures the company meets its legal obligations under the Saskatchewan Health and Safety Act (one of the country's strictest). In a non-industrial workplace, this is not an onerous task, but she still has to do such things as perform regular noise-level checks and hearing tests for employees in the print shop. (Kushnir Pekrul is a certified screening audiologist.) Similarly, she ensures compliance with federal hazardous-waste regulations, notably by overseeing use and storage of chemicals in the in-house audiovisual department.

Occupational-health nurses got their start in the U.S. mining industry. In Canada, the first corporation to have nurses on staff to ensure the health of their employees was Eaton's, which began the practice more than a century ago. It's a job that varies greatly, depending on context. In the automotive industry, nurses worry about fire safety and preventing machine injuries; in the meat-packing industry, they stitch people up and try to change processes to minimize knife wounds; and, in the white-collar world, ergonomics and preventing heart disease top the list.

Kushnir Pekrul says occupational-health nursing is a little-known specialty, even in the nursing profession. And hospitals, institutions that are among those most in need of a health-promotion service and that stand to be the most direct beneficiaries, do not tend to employ occupational-health nurses themselves. (Ironically, nurses are close to the top of the list in terms of sick days taken; they average 12 sick days annually, significantly more than the 7.8 days claimed by the average Canadian worker.)

The difficulty is that occupational-health nursing is a solitary profession (usually one nurse per company) so there is little research done into the benefits. Similarly, the Canadian health-care system, which conducts elaborate tracking of medical procedures, does not do the same for preventive medicine. In the United States, on the other hand, many companies have ties to health-management organizations (HMOs), and they do elaborate tracking of wellness measures. Because of the financial benefits of keeping employees healthy, they also offer a lot of incentives. For example, white-collar employees in the United States who do not make a health claim during the year can be eligible for gifts, such as a set of golf clubs or free plane tickets.

Kushnir Pekrul says there is a fascinating paradox there that needs to be explored, the fact that private enterprise has caught on to the benefits of health promotion while the public system continues to pay little more than lip service to the idea. "Everything we do in our health centre is consistent with all the good stuff in the Canadian health system and all the stuff it should be doing. Here we are in private enterprise, and we've embraced a wellness model and nurse-managed primary health-care model," she says.

"As a nurse, I truly believe in our public health-care system, but I'm always struggling with the real philosophical dichotomy that arises from reality. If it's so cost-effective to do this—and it is or the company wouldn't to it—then why doesn't every worker in Canada have access to this kind of help? If it's going to save the health system billions of dollars every year, why isn't there an occupational-health nurse in every workplace?"

Part Five
MENTAL HEALTH

The Untouchables

At some point in their lives, one in four Canadians will struggle with addiction or mental illness. Despite the pervasiveness of such conditions, there is widespread fear and apprehension about them, and there is also silence. Deadly silence.

Critical Care looks at nursing throughout the life cycle. Part Five, however, focuses on nurses who work with people with psychiatric and developmental disabilities, as well as addictions, of all ages. Mental illness cuts across every category of society. It affects young and old, women and men, rich and poor.

Depression is the leading cause of disability in the world. It costs the Canadian economy more than $12 billion annually in lost productivity, and it is the leading cause of absenteeism. Substance abuse is even more damaging, costing the economy an estimated $18 billion a year.

Mental illness and addiction also have repercussions that extend far beyond those of many other diseases. The social and economic consequences of being labelled "retarded," "schizo," or "junkie" are devastating. So, while people will talk openly about their struggles with breast cancer and heart disease—an important part of the healing process—they will not do so after a bout with depression or prescription-drug addiction.

Stereotypes and prejudices are deeply rooted. The mentally ill are often viewed as morally weak, dangerous, and incontrovertibly crazy. As a result, they are too often denied understanding, compassion, and care. A huge proportion of the mentally ill are condemned not only to struggling alone, but to marginalization, to poverty, and to institutionalization (increasingly in prisons, not treatment facilities).

The nurses featured here, who work daily with the mentally ill and those with developmental disabilities, care deeply, and at times heroically, for their patients. It is not a coincidence that psychiatric nurses, particularly those toiling in the community during these mean times, are among the most vocal and strong-minded women in the profession. They are not only caregivers, but activists.

Cathy Crowe, from her base on Queen Street West in Toronto, has become one of the most respected and feared (at least by foot-dragging politicians) defenders of the homeless. As a public-health nurse, she long ago realized that a home is a prerequisite to good health. Without a roof over your head, you cannot eat right, you cannot avoid disease, you cannot work, you cannot be an active member of society. Across the country, on Vancouver's troubled east side, Liz Evans came to a similar realization. Her clientele of "unhousables" is a disparate group of square pegs having a difficult time finding a place in a conservative society that wants everyone to fit into a round hole of conformity.

Evans and Crowe are following in the footsteps of public-health pioneers who created programs such as needle exchanges, methadone programs, and mobile soup kitchens. What is remarkable is their ability to be non-judgmental, to pursue harm-reduction strategies in the face of much negative reaction, because, ultimately, they realize all society will benefit. De-institutionalization in the 1970s and 1980s was, in theory, a wonderful concept. Many, many people with psychiatric and developmental disabilities did not belong in hospitals. They were returned to the community. But too many were abandoned there, without appropriate and necessary supports. Where programs do exist to help them pick up the pieces, nurses are almost certain to be at the forefront.

The urban homeless who roam the streets of big cities, trapped in their addictions and turning to prostitution and crime to survive, are the most visible mentally ill in Canada today. But they are not the extreme. An even tinier minority are the criminally insane, those whose disease leads them to maim and to murder. Kerry Ferguson deals with these patients in her role as a nurse at St. Thomas Psychiatric Hospital in southwestern Ontario. She cares for some of society's most reviled, people who are being assessed to determine if they are fit to stand trial. There is obviously a need for such institutions, which, despite their grim reputations, are far preferable to the prison system for people with mental illness, who get no appropriate treatment in the latter.

Community nurse Christine McCarthy deals with another segment of the population entirely, providing education for group-home workers and the developmentally disabled themselves, over a vast territory. This is one of the success stories of the mental-health field, seeing people once labelled as retarded and hopeless integrate into and blossom in the community.

McCarthy and Ferguson, you will note, are not in the least bit frightened by the mentally ill and the developmentally disabled. They see beyond the surface differences, beyond the stereotypes. They recognize that only 4 per cent of violence in society is attributable to people with psychiatric disabilities. The reality is that, when those suffering from mental illness are violent, it is usually towards themselves. There are almost 4,000 suicides in the country annually—11 per day—with more than half of them among those suffering from depression.

It is important to remember that most people with mental illness and addictions lead active, productive lives. They are work colleagues, fellow churchgoers, the woman pushing a stroller to the park, the man laughing over coffee at the restaurant. Some of Canada's top business leaders require regular treatment to keep their depression in check, as do gifted artists, hard-working labourers, and nurses. Leading politicians attend Alcoholics Anonymous meetings, alongside decorated soldiers and schoolteachers.

Anna-Liisa Dean works with those who are lucky enough to be admitted to the Homewood Health Centre, where they can get state-of-the-art treatment for their addictions and psychiatric illnesses. In her work, she deals with a clientele drawn from a cross-section of society. Overrepresented in the mix, not surprisingly, are health-care professionals, including nurses. Nursing is stressful, isolating work that, while offering great personal rewards, can exacerbate problems such as addiction and depression.

When people don't know where to turn for help, they invariably end up in the emergency room. Proof that mental illness has reached epidemic proportions in society is that virtually every emergency room now has a psychiatric nurse on staff. Fred Haines performs this role in Saskatoon, but the experience is remarkably similar in big and small towns alike, with emergency rooms at times looking like mini psychiatric wards of old.

While governments brag about closing psychiatric hospitals, regular hospitals have simply absorbed much of the clientele by adding psychiatric wards and expanding their emergency-room programs. Schizophrenia, for example, requires greater use of hospital beds than any other medical or surgical condition. And one-quarter of the 34 million hospital days paid for by our publicly funded medical system each year are used to treat people with mental illness.

Research has shown that for every dollar spent on treating addictions and mental illness, society saves up to $7 in legal and social costs. If this section demonstrates anything, it is that investing in nurses pays dividends not only immediately, but over the long term. The work of nurses ministering to homeless people in back alleys is as important as the work of those in high-tech hospitals, caring for burned-out professionals. And what they have in common is that they are redefining the boundaries of health care, and the definition of nursing.

Home Street Home — Cathy Crowe

"I'm a street nurse. My specialty is working with the homeless," Cathy Crowe says, pausing before uttering the kicker. "It's obscene that in city as wealthy as Toronto, in a country like Canada, that such a specialty even exists."

Having worked in Toronto's inner city for the past twenty-seven years, Crowe is currently a nurse-practitioner operating a small clinic at Queen West Community Health Centre. She also has regular clinic hours at a number of facilities in the neighbourhood, where the homeless congregate, and does "house calls" to shelters and squats where other health professionals will not go.

Crowe never leaves the office without her ever-present knap-sack. Its contents offer insight on her work, and her clientele: Ensure (a nutritional supplement for the malnourished), vitamins, antibiotic creams, antifungals, dressing supplies, Tylenol, surgical gloves, sunscreen, bus tickets, and bottled water.

A short walk from the glittering towers of Bay Street, the opulent waterfront condominiums, and the luxurious SkyDome, thousands of people are going hungry, blistering their feet as they wander the streets, being consumed by infectious disease and crushed by hopelessness because they have no place to live. Crowe sees the city's homeless as residents of a giant, quasi-invisible refugee camp. Like refugees, they suffer emotional deprivation, a constant assault on their immune systems, and ever-looming phys-ical threats (risk of violence, sexual asssault, police brutality), and a shockingly high death rate. "Medically, I can't do a lot. What is needed here is a political solution to the underlying problem of homelessness," Crowe says.

Contrary to popular belief, most of her clientele are not old winos. Many homeless are now in their thirties, not people who have severe psychiatric or drug-abuse problems (those come later, as a coping mechanism), but, rather, ordinary working folk who suffered a sharp reversal—job loss, broken marriage, sexual abuse—and got caught in a downward spiral that left them penni-less and on the streets. "I've met a lot of business people on the streets—a chiropractor, even a nurse. Nobody can be smug, because it's a disaster that any one of us could be dragged into," Crowe notes.

She will see about twenty patients during a two-hour clinic. Most have ulcerated or frostbitten feet that she treats with ointment and a new pair of socks. Many suffer from heat stroke, scurvy, and tuberculosis (about 40 per cent of her clientele have been exposed to the bacterium). There are stitches and broken bones to be tended to, and souls so battered that they cannot be repaired. Several times a week, the nurse will rush down to the lobby to tend to a patient who could not make it to the second-floor clinic, a victim of overdose, stabbing, or starvation.

Between two and four homeless people die each week in Toronto, most of them meeting a violent end, with murder and suicide topping the list. So marginalized is her clientele that, until Crowe started, nobody even bothered counting the dead. "I'm a community-health nurse. I shouldn't have to deal with this volume of death," Crowe says. "And as a society, we cannot accept this volume of homeless people."

Because of the enormity of the problems she sees, Crowe has shifted increasingly from "direct service" to political advocacy. But the clinics, the street nurse says, are essential for keeping her grounded, and for giving her the legitimacy to speak out. "Doing the clinics fuels the political activism. I couldn't do one without the other," she says. "People trust me and speak frankly to me. And I speak frankly on their behalf. I think that's why I'm listened to."

Homelessness, for Crowe, is one of the biggest public-health issues in Canada today. There are an estimated 200,000 homeless in Canada. A task force led by Anne Golden, president of the United Way of Metropolitan Toronto, found that there are as many as 80,000 people in Toronto who are homeless or at risk of being so in the near future. Since 1998, Crowe has been calling the problem a national disaster, and that has finally attracted the attention of the public and politicians.

The approach came to her, Crowe says, when she experienced a "nursing epiphany" while watching television-news coverage of the 1998 ice storm. Like many Canadians, she was shocked to see the extent of damage and the number of displaced people, and was going to volunteer her services as a nurse. After all, for the previous eleven years she had been working in crowded drop-ins and shelters, often alone and without running water, adequate light, or proper supplies; she could certainly handle an emergency.

"But then I realized that the images on television that had moved me were the daily circumstances of homeless people's lives. I was overcome by grief and nausea as this truth hit home. The comparison to the ice storm was a painful reminder to me that homeless people, no matter where they are in Canada, quite simply have no home, no central heart of support or base. Many have had no home for years."

Crowe, like most nurses of her era, was trained at a hospital, St. Michael's Hospital in Toronto. After graduation, she worked a nine-to-five job doing cardiac stress testing at a private clinic, but was looking for a challenge. One night she watched a TVOntario documentary about South Riverdale Community Health Centre, and, on a whim, applied for a job. She got a taste of street nursing working in Toronto's most downtrodden neighbourhood, Regent Park, then went to work for Street Health, a dynamic nurse-run health agency for the homeless. Paralleling her day job was her increased community involvement, in groups such as Nurses for Social Responsibility, which spoke out against nuclear arms and the death penalty and in favour of reproductive choice, and the Toronto Coalition Against Homelessness, which staged a high-profile public inquiry into the death of street people in Toronto.

During the ice storm, she began rallying others in the community to her new approach and, by June 1998 they had formed the Toronto Disaster Relief Committee. The group, in a declaration that was issued with much fanfare a few months later, called homelessness an "epidemic which no civilized society can tolerate," and called for resources to be mobilized as they would be for an earthquake or hurricane, including short-term "rescue" measures (namely, more and better shelters), and for the addition of 1 per cent to government housing budgets.

As the initiative picked up steam and went national, Crowe

found herself drawn into an endless series of meetings. After a full day's work on the streets, she still finds that most of her evenings feature some kind of meeting, either at City Hall or with community groups.

In the process, Crowe became a recognizable media figure, and is quoted regularly in news stories. This is unusual for nurses, who are often forbidden by their employers from taking public stands. (The Queen West Community Health Centre is funded by the Ontario government, and Crowe says that, while she has never been muzzled, she is always careful to identify herself as speaking for the Toronto Disaster Relief Committee, not the centre.)

The committee, she says, made a conscious effort to have street nurses as spokespersons because they have an almost inherent credibility. But what does all the advocacy have to do with community health and nursing?

Crowe's response is immediate and adamant: "Housing is one of the prerequisites for health. You can't eat well, you can't sleep well, you can't care for your health, if you don't have a roof over your head. It's basic. And as a community-health nurse, I have a responsibility to speak out when I see the makings of an acute disaster."

Crowe also believes that it is a basic tenet of nursing to reach out to those in need, regardless of their station in life, and to advocate for patients when they are discriminated against. "I keep doing it because I believe I'm making a difference not only on the streets, but on the political landscape. Just imagine how much more of a difference we could make if we made a concerted effort as a society to eradicate homelessness."

The Unhousables—Liz Evans

Saturday morning in February. Vancouver's downtown east side looks even grimier than usual under winter clouds and a chilly wind. The dilapidated Portland Hotel would not warrant a second look, except for the young woman who has dashed through the doorway to escape the rain.

In sharp contrast to her surroundings, Liz Evans is beaming, wearing leopard-print tights, with a chic black skirt and sweater. Smiling and greeting virtually everybody in the lobby by name, she bounds up the stairs to her office, a ramshackle room featuring a computer, piles of paper, and an impressive array of security monitors.

Evans may look like a carefree young woman, but, as the associate executive director of Portland Hotel Society, which provides housing for the unhousable, she has an unenviable job. The group began in 1990, operating out of an old rooming house. It now runs a ten-storey facility with eighty-six rooms, the New Portland Hotel, and manages four other facilities with almost 200 more beds.

The folks sprawled around the lobby of the Old Portland are probably the most down-and-out collection of individuals you will find anywhere in Canada. They are, in the jargon of the health-and-welfare system, the "multidiagnosed," people with a frightening array of health problems, both physical and psychological. There are hard-core junkies, chronic alcoholics, hardened criminals, victims of sexual abuse, fading sex-trade workers, the gravely mentally ill. Any number of them can, at any given moment, be teetering dangerously close to overdose or grappling loudly with their demons, never mind the litany of physical ailments: complications from HIV and AIDS; hepatitis A, B, and C; tuberculosis; endocarditis (a bacterial infection that damages the heart); septicaemia (blood poisoning); cirrhosis; pneumonia; cellulitis (a skin disease); malnutrition; and the complications from wounds. During Evans's first day on the job, a man was beaten to death with a baseball bat outside the front door. Their average life expectancy: age 38.

The residents of Portland Hotel have been banned from every other shelter, drop-in, and hospice in the city for their violent, antisocial behaviour. They have been cast aside by society as its ultimate losers. Evans is their den mother. "The shelters and the rooming houses have a lot of rules, and they end up kicking people out on the streets. When they have nowhere else to go, they come here. We have a mandate to not evict people. We fit around people rather than impose rules on them."

The philosophy here is harm reduction. If a resident is psychotic and smashes the windows in his room, they are replaced with Plexiglas. If an intravenous drug user is not interested in detox, clean needles are provided. If a chronic alcoholic wants to get drunk, you try to ensure he will drink cheap wine instead of Listerine.

"By the time they get to Portland, they have been circulated through the system many times. They have failed repeatedly and the system has failed them repeatedly. We pretty well let them be. We don't pass judgment on people, we provide care. We're the ultimate pragmatists, I guess," Evans says.

The Portland Hotel's approach infuriates many law-and-order types and it disgusts some other social-service agencies, but it is hard to deny that, for this particular clientele, it works. In fact, the project has attracted the interest of public-health officials around the world and funding from government and private donors, not because it creates miracles, but in large part because of the cost savings it generates.

A psychiatrist at St. Paul's Hospital calculated the cost to the health and justice system of two of Portland's residents prior to their arrival, and the results were shocking. The two, who were frequently arrested for petty crimes and made regular visits to emergency rooms, ran up costs of $2.8 million over a three-year period, just in 9-1-1 responses and Emergency admissions (the researcher didn't factor in justice-system costs).

After six months at Portland, where they were allowed to deal with issues at their own pace, and where they were not clashing repeatedly with the authorities, the two were leading far more stable lives. One is still an addict, but takes methadone instead of heroin, and the overdoses and violent outbursts are way down. She has required very few emergency calls over the past five years. The other, who used to get high and run naked through malls, has graduated with a high-school equivalency and is now studying for a college degree by correspondence.

Evans is a pragmatist. She does not try to glorify Portland, admitting it is barely one step above the street. "We recognize that this place is crappy, but it's better than nothing—and the alternative for our residents is nothing," she says.

Having a roof over their heads, however modest, allows residents to get medical care. The stability is also one of the most effective means of preventing medical episodes that are harmful and costly to the system. This clientele frequently visits hospital emergency rooms, with drug-related problems and violence-related injuries. Left untreated (because most are thrown out of hospitals and clinics in short order), they are vectors for disease transmission. Epidemiologists know that getting to this population, which tends to be transient and difficult to treat, is the key to limiting the outbreak of infectious diseases.

Portland has three clinics a week, with a doctor and two public-health nurses. Most of their work is wound care, testing for infectious disease and coordinating antiretroviral treatment for those infected with HIV. The housing project also has a full-time care coordinator, who is also a nurse. This is in addition to Evans, whose role is largely administrative.

Still, she says her background as a psychiatric emergency nurse is invaluable. Evans does a lot of assessment—for example, to determine the gravity of a psychotic episode or an overdose. She does a lot of counselling and hand-holding, given the volatile lives many residents lead and the fact that most have cut all ties with family and friends. Increasingly, she is also getting involved in palliative care.

"Many choose to die here in the shitty old hotel because they get kicked out of hospice, or they don't feel comfortable there. There is this strange notion that, as people are about to die, we have to dress them up and put them in a clean, sterile institution. It's so hypocritical because nobody gives a damn about them when they're alive," Evans says, rubbing her tired eyes.

The education of workers, for which she is also partly responsible, is unlike anything a nurse-educator would do in a hospital.

With more than 90 per cent of Portland residents taking medications at least daily (with few of them prone to compliance), and most of them on an Ensure weight-gain program, staff really have to know their meds and nutrition. They also need training on how to deal with people with mental illness, substance-abuse problems, infectious diseases, and palliative-care needs—well over half the residents are infected with HIV-AIDS, and many are in the end stages. The work is so emotionally and physically demanding that workers at the shelter have a four-day week. They also receive ongoing counselling and training.

There is an on-site needle exchange and, because of the potential for violence, all workers carry a panic button and are trained in self-defence. Yet, because of the non-confrontational approach, there is only about one violent attack every two years, a better record that most emergency rooms. "And don't forget to mention plumbing," Evans quips. "Everybody here has to know how to unclog a toilet."

The medical, self-defence, and home-maintenance training is all inextricable from the political training. Staff have lengthy discussions on what it means to do good in society, and they study the history of the poor and the ethics of care. Because most Canadians are sheltered from the urban underbelly, most workers have a "crisis of enlightenment" that gets them more socially engaged. Evans can be found at a lot of demonstrations, and has become a leading advocate of decriminalization of drugs, saying the money spent on enforcement and imprisonment would be better spent on social housing.

She readily admits to being "so naïve" when she took the job at Portland, but does not regret for a moment leaving the institutional setting (she had worked at Vancouver General Hospital and Royal Ottawa Hospital) for the community. "I left the hospital because I saw people during brief psychotic episodes, and then released them back into nothing. I never felt like I was providing care. You have to care for people in a holistic way; you have to look at the whole person, their background and their environment. You have to understand the social determinants of health and the practical reality of their lives. You have to adapt," Evans says.

In her view, modern nursing is obsessed with professionalism and rigid categorization, and needs to put the focus back on caring. Evans let her active-practice licence lapse—in large part because renewal was expensive and the pay at Portland is lousy—and is now fighting to get it back (principally because she would like to do a master's but needs an active licence to do so). At one point, the Registered Nurses Association of B.C. was mulling over whether or not to classify what Evans does as nursing. The formal answer has not yet come, but in the meantime the association awarded Evans its Health Advocacy Award, and lauded the groundbreaking work she is doing.

"I deal with sick and dying people every minute of every day. I provide health care in the context of where people live. And I fight and advocate on their behalf. If that's not nursing, I don't know what is."

The Cuckoo's Nest—Kerry Ferguson

St. Thomas Psychiatric Hospital is the kind of place that features prominently in nightmares. Medieval-looking from the outside, it has that haunting institutional look on the inside, with endless green, echoing hallways. Waiting for the door to swing open and for a severe-looking psychiatric nurse to appear, clad in a starched white uniform, one cannot help but think of a certain movie.

"Oh, I love *One Flew Over the Cuckoo's Nest*," says Kerry Ferguson. "It's a *great* movie—but it's fiction. The patients say it to you all the time, 'Nurse Ratched, Nurse Ratched.' But it's just a joke." Ferguson doesn't even wear white, opting for scrubs. And her shoes are rubber-soled, so there's no menacing clicking when she walks the halls.

There are no feces splattered on the wall, no lobotomy scars, no electroshock room, no patients staring catatonically at the TV. "And, you know what? In thirteen years working here, I've never seen a straitjacket," she adds.

In fact, the most frightening aspect of psychiatric hospitals today is their emptiness. St. Thomas, one of ten psychiatric facilities in Ontario, was once home to 2,500 patients. Now, it houses 203. The province will undoubtedly follow the lead of others and close its psychiatric institutions entirely. (British Columbia was the first to do so, about a decade ago.)

This is a mixed blessing. There were abuses in the past, people locked away who could have functioned well within the community, with adequate supports. But the pendulum has swung too far. To save money, people with chronic psychiatric problems are dumped into the general population without the help they need to maintain a decent standard of living. There are simply not enough psychiatric nurses in the community setting to keep pace, and it is not a constituency with any political clout.

"I don't see the hospital being here much longer, certainly not until the end of my career, so I'll probably end up in the community," Ferguson says. "But I know it's a lot harder out there. They just don't have the resources."

The constant threat of job loss is one of the biggest stresses of the job. The hospital has already been merged, administratively, with London Psychiatric Hospital, and all the institutions will soon come under the control of St. Joseph's Health Centre. Ferguson says staff have been waiting for years for the axe to fall and "it wears on you." In an era of cutbacks, it makes no sense to operate a giant hospital that is practically empty.

Ferguson could also end up working in a prison, where all too many of the mentally ill end up, having traded one institution for another that is far worse because treatment is virtually non-existent.

Her job, in the forensic assessment unit, is already as much part of the criminal-justice system as it is the health system. All the patients, most of them under the age of 40, have been charged with criminal offences, and are there by court order to determine if they are fit to stand trial or if they should be deemed "not criminally responsible."

Nurses interact as they would in a hospital setting, dispensing medication and operating as a sounding board for patients, except that meticulous notes must be taken, and anything patients say can be used against them at their court hearings.

Another complication in a program where people are sent against their will is that many refuse to cooperate in their treatment—namely, they refuse to take medication. At one time, they could be forced, but now that the Mental Health Act has been reformed, almost anyone has the right to refuse treatment.

For a long-time nurse like Ferguson, this is a travesty. "I think it's great that people who can make sound decisions have more rights. But I've fought the Mental Health Act because it hurts those who need the most help. It takes a lot more time to help people now because they refuse their meds and they refuse to participate in programs. They just smoke and sleep all day. All we've done is give them the right to not get treatment, to not get better, when they're not thinking straight," she says dejectedly.

When Ferguson began at the hospital in 1986, patients were still assigned manual labour on the sprawling grounds (and they were paid a minimal wage), and they had far more regimented treatment programs. "They got better a lot faster. Today we have much better medication [a lot of the worst side effects have been attenuated] but we don't do as well with lots of people," she says.

Ferguson works almost exclusively nights, from 7:00 P.M. to 7:00 A.M.; five shifts one week, two the next, and she gets every second weekend off. The shift starts with snacks, medication, and showering for the patients, and then conversation. There are sixteen beds on the unit, generally with a ratio of two men for every woman. Each nurse is assigned a primary patient and a couple of other patients.

"To an outsider, it looks like we just sit around and chat, but understanding the illness and being able to talk about it is an essential part of the treatment," Ferguson says. "Sometimes it can get heavy, when they want to talk about mental illness or what they have done. Lots of them don't have any family support or any friends after years of mental illness. The nurse is really the only person they have left."

After lights out at 11:00 P.M., nurses write up reports and do crisis management. Patients who are being monitored for threat of suicide and who are in restraints (and there are usually at least a couple) have to be watched constantly. Rounds are hourly. Because of their underlying illness or medication, many patients have trouble sleeping. Psychotic episodes are not uncommon.

For Ferguson, the worst thing that happens are the fights between patients. Staff get regular training in self-defence, holds, and use of restraints.* She has chronic back problems from years of "wrestling" but says violence is not a major problem, even with the criminally insane.

"Over all the years, I can only think of three or four I've really been afraid of—you could just see the danger in their eyes. But I've never been attacked here. Geriatrics is a lot worse than Psych. An old farmer hit me once; he was big and strong and it really hurt," she says.

The majority of patients in forensic assessment have committed crimes related directly to their mental illness, such as assault, uttering death threats, and destruction of property. There is the occasional killer. Many are charged with break-and-enter or robbery, crimes often perpetrated to feed a drug habit. There are a multitude of diagnoses, but chronic schizophrenia, manic depression, and anxiety depression are most common. "But we don't see the real psychopaths anymore. They go right to prison and don't really get any help," she says.

There are, of course, frustrations. Ferguson knows of one patient who had been admitted to the psychiatric hospital fifty-eight times in the past decade. The irony of de-institutionalization

---

* The most common form of restraint today is wrist-to-waist restraint, which allows enough mobility for patients to smoke and drink coffee, but not enough for them to do serious harm to themselves or others. If a patient is truly disturbed, nurses will use double restraints, ankle-to-ankle. But straitjackets have not been in use for years.

is that, for a core group of the mentally ill, it is harder than ever to get out of the system. They just keep passing through a revolving door, circling from the community to jail and back to the hospital without ever getting consistent treatment.

Ferguson is frustrated, too, that, despite the much more visible presence of the mentally ill in society, the public still harbours prejudices and really does not have even a basic understanding of psychiatric illness. "People are smug about mental illness. They say 'I'm too strong, it won't happen to me.' What I say is that any one of us could be in here tomorrow. I've been a psych nurse my whole career, and I can tell you: It's not us and them. It's all just us."

Tearing Down the Walls — Christine McCarthy

The Oxford Regional Centre in Woodstock, Ontario, closed its doors on March 31, 1996. It now awaits the wrecker's ball, a boarded-up, dilapidated reminder of a time, not long ago, when many people with developmental disabilities were locked away, hidden from public view.

Those once called the "retarded" are certainly more visible, but their freedom has come at a price. The jobs of thousands of nurses who cared for them have disappeared, and only a fraction of those nurses are working in the community. While supports in most communities are clearly inadequate, people with developmental disabilities are well served compared with those with psychiatric illnesses.

The Canadian Association for Community Living and other community groups have been powerful advocates for de-institutionalization, in addition to providing on-the-ground support. Today, they continue to push for improvements in the system, including demands for more community nurses to serve the unique needs of this important minority within the population.

Christine McCarthy has followed this evolution closely, and has a vested interest in the changes. A former nurse at Oxford Regional

Centre, she now works for Regional Support Associates, a group of health consultants that assists the developmentally disabled in southwestern Ontario. The private company has a contract with Woodstock General Hospital, which, in turn, gets funding for the program from the provincial Ministry of Community and Social Services. (This is an example of how many nurses are, increasingly, on the government payroll in an indirect manner.)

The group of fifteen consultants provides service in seven counties, a vast geographic area. McCarthy is the only nurse on a team of physicians, psychologists, counsellors, and behaviour therapists, all of whom used to work in the institutional setting.

McCarthy's principal role is that of educator. Most people with severe developmental disabilities live in group homes, and she does much of her work with employees of these small facilities. The main goal is to teach workers—who range from high-school students to highly educated professionals—how health issues can affect behaviour, in the belief that early intervention will prevent health problems. "Lots of the members of this population are non-verbal, so direct communication is poor, or non-existent. Your interpretation of their behaviour is the key to understanding the state of their health," McCarthy says.

For example, a mentally handicapped person may, if he has an earache, not point to the spot of the pain, but hit his head repeatedly on the wall. "It's a bit like a puzzle with some pieces missing. The clients give you signals, but you have to figure out what they mean," she says.

For a public-health system, dedicating specialized resources such as nursing care to this population pays big dividends. Many people with developmental disabilities have chronic bowel problems, due to an oversized colon that causes severe difficulties in terms of motility. In fact, many still die young from bowel obstructions. McCarthy does teaching in group homes that includes diet tips, how to give enemas and insert suppositories, and how to do charting that allows early detection of problems.

While it is appropriate for much of this work to be done by

group-home workers, there are times when she is disturbed by the off-loading that is taking place in the name of cost savings. At one point, McCarthy was asked to teach workers to give intramuscular injections, a task usually reserved for a nurse. "I really had to draw the line because I would be putting my nursing licence on the line," she says. But pressures like this are being continually exerted on nurses, particularly those with little job security.

McCarthy says the consultant role is different from a bedside job in the way you judge your impact and get feedback. "In the centre, you saw the results of what you were doing immediately—or as immediately as they come, in this field. Now, the reward comes in an indirect way, when people come up in a group home, shake your hand, and say: 'I hear you do good work.' You realize that the teaching you do is going to have a positive impact on people for years to come."

The days when people with developmental disabilities were routinely sterilized are behind us (though most institutions prescribe the Pill to women of child-bearing age because sexual contact is not uncommon between patients). In the community, a public-health nurse plays an important role in relationship counselling and in teaching about sexuality and birth control. "People get all preachy about this, but the practical reality is that you need a good support system in place if you're going to have effective birth control," McCarthy says. Above all, couples need someone with whom they are comfortable discussing such personal issues, and the nurse tends to fill that function.

People with disabilities are also extremely vulnerable to fraud artists and sexual abusers. "So teaching about birth control tends to stray into areas like street safety and personal space. But it all makes for a healthier individual," she says.

When McCarthy worked at Oxford Regional Centre, she ran a small health clinic within the institution, one that dealt with bowel problems, birth control, insulin injections, and fractures (this population also has a very high incidence of skull fractures due to falls, often related to seizures). But in a structured environment, the patients led sheltered, empty lives with few surprises. From a nursing point of view, it was fairly predictable and not too challenging. McCarthy says that institutions were a magnet for people looking for civil-service jobs, but those working in the community are far more dedicated to their clients and engaged in the issues. "It's such a different kind of nursing out in the community. You really have to think on your feet—which is really what good nursing is all about anyhow," she says.

And McCarthy insists that life is far better for her clients: "Lots of the old staff predicted the patients would die in the community, but, for the most part, the DH [developmentally handicapped] population is flourishing. It's not always easy, but they're out there, they're making choices and they're living. From my perspective, there has been a great improvement in their health and their quality of life." Yet lingering effects of the long-standing policy of institutionalization remain, chief among them isolation and social stigmatization. People were put away for so long in hospitals that they lost all family support and never learned the basics of community living.

The move to the community has also been a professional rebirth for McCarthy, but it has not altered her job security. For six years at Oxford Regional Centre, she lived under the constant threat of layoff—an experience many nurses in smaller hospitals know all too well—as rumours swirled and staff dwindled around her. But life in private enterprise is no less precarious than it was on the public payroll. Due to the convoluted funding arrangement, McCarthy doesn't have any permanence, any holidays (she gets holiday pay), or a pension plan. "I don't even have a contract. I have a promise. And the funding to back up that promise is on a wing and a prayer," she says with a chuckle. "It's like any job in nursing today: the job could be gone tomorrow."

Travelling about with a laptop and a cellular phone, she has a lot of freedom, though the travel demands (almost 40,000 kilometres a year) are wearing. But there are benefits. "I work four days a week, straight days. I think a lot of nurses would kill for those hours," she says.

The shift to the community and to consulting has also left McCarthy confident that she will never be wanting for work. "I think lots of nurses get comfortable in their jobs and they don't realize the opportunities that are out there."

The Spectrum of Calamities—Anna-Liisa Dean

Every nurse has a blood-curdling tale about a shift from hell. Anna-Liisa Dean's kicked off with a loud argument involving a belligerent co-worker. Rounds revealed a particularly demanding group of clients. A patient on suicide watch slipped out of the hospital. Following closely on his heels was a second patient, suffering from severe withdrawal. The second patient soon returned, under police escort. Later during the night, he broke out again, wriggling through a tiny bathroom window, jumping from the roof, and breaking an ankle. When he finally returned, transferred in an ambulance from another hospital, the man jumped off the stretcher and punched one of Dean's co-workers (and not the obnoxious one she was bickering with throughout the ordeal). Then, thankfully, the suicidal patient was found unharmed. All this in addition to the regular demands of a twelve-hour shift working with dozens of patients with severe addictions.

"That was definitely my worst shift, but, at the best of times, this work can be emotionally draining and physically exhausting," says Dean, a nurse at Homewood Health Centre, a privately owned but publicly funded institution in Guelph, Ontario. "It's a nursing job that really spans the spectrum of human calamities."

Alcoholism, drug abuse (from prescription sleeping pills through to heroin), pathological gambling, nicotine addiction, and sexual dependency are the principal reasons people seek treatment, but what predominates is a combination, often with concurrent psychiatric disorders or deep psychological traumas. The age range is broad, but most are between the ages of 30 and 40, when addictions have really begun to catch up with them. There are about as many women as men. "The patients we see vary, but, if they have something in common, it's that they have done a lot of damage to themselves and to their loved ones, and that alcohol is very much a strain throughout," Dean says.

She has experienced the heartbreak that many families know all too well, because of an alcoholic brother. A successful entrepreneur, he lost his business, saw his marriage dissolve, and suffered severe health problems because of drinking, but she still had a lot of trouble getting him into treatment. "It really personalizes the job. I know how much damage he has done to his life, and I understand the family perspective, the frustration they feel," she says. But her brother is now in his third year of sobriety, Dean says proudly, and that is inspiring when working with others.

Homewood treats about 2,000 people a year for various addictions. There are 312 beds, 86 of them in the addictions unit (there are also programs for victims of sexual abuse, traumatic-stress recovery, depression/anxiety, eating disorders, and psychogeriatrics), and there is rarely a free bed at the renowned institution.*

The program lasts six weeks; it has a standardized core but is individualized to the needs of each patient. During the week, there are six nurses on duty. Because the addictions program is quite regimented, so is the work of the nurses who provide the core care. One will be assigned to stripping beds, another to laundry, one to moving patients from room to room, one to new admissions, and another to overseeing medications. At the same time, each will be assigned specific patients to watch over.

A typical day begins at 7:00 A.M. with a prerounds group meeting involving nurses, doctors, and counsellors. There, they decide on assignments, and specific interventions for clients. Then there are more formal rounds.

For patients, the day usually starts with medication to help them deal with withdrawal. There is breakfast and a walk. Then another

---

* Homewood has been operating since 1883.

round of medication (it is not unusual for patients to receive Valium as frequently as hourly), and meditation. Nurses are constantly taking vital signs and reassessing patients because withdrawal can be physically punishing and, in the early days, the danger of seizures is ever present. The Homewood philosophy is that addiction has a biological or genetic basis, and treatment is proferred according to a medical model. "Addiction is not a choice and you don't need a kick in the pants. Far from it. You need support," Dean says.

Much of the mornings are taken up with meetings of groups such as Alcoholics Anonymous or Narcotics Anonymous, or smoking-cessation programs. During this time, nurses have to complete their assigned tasks, do a lot of charting, and spend a lot of time processing orders, such as for referrals and medication.

Throughout the day, there is time set aside for patients' journaling, visiting, and socializing. One of the key roles of nurses is to promote interaction between patients (and to step in as peacemakers when edgy people get into arguments and fights). Those with privileges go shopping at the mall, or engage in sports at Homewood's recreation facilities.

"Isolation is a big part of addiction, so socializing is an important component of our program," Dean says. Another essential role for nurses is providing feedback. Each patient must check in at least twice a day with a nurse. There is a physical assessment, because many addicts have ailments brought about by their abuse. It is also a time to determine how well patients are doing psychologically, to assess how they are coping with the rigours of recovery, and to cut them short when they are engaging in drug-seeking activities, and the lying and deception that go along with it. "It's like a firefighter role: you try to douse the problems early before they get out of control," Dean says.

After supper, patients usually have another support-group meeting (two or three a day is common), and after 9:00 P.M. they can retire to either the movie lounge or the sports lounge. The two-TV system, devised by nurses, defused the main source of tension in the ward—who controlled the remote control. But, even in leisure time, nurses are constantly vigilant. They must approve movies, to avoid those that would act as triggers to people battling addictions (*Leaving Las Vegas* comes readily to mind), and they must also keep those with gambling problems out of the sports lounge.

On the weekend, when Dean, a part-timer, does the bulk of her work, there is a single nurse on the ward. The nursing focus is also dramatically different. Many patients head home to their families, but those who are most unstable tend to stay. They have a lot more time with nurses, who will spend many hours talking, primarily working with them on planning and focus so they can complete the program successfully.

The listening, the one-on-one caring for someone in need, is rewarding, she says, but it is also very taxing. "It's hard to hear a lot of the stuff, the sex abuse especially. They are very needy clients, and it takes a lot out of you." The other challenge is making sure to give attention to those making progress, not just those who speak loudest. "As a nurse, you never want a client to think: 'She was too busy, she didn't have time.' You have to try and be there for those who really need you," she says.

A number of patients, however, are not in the recovery program willingly. Some are there "on forms" (under the provisions of the Mental Health Act), while others are there grudgingly, usually because of an ultimatum from a spouse or an employer. "People are not necessarily here willingly or ready for the program. They have to get past the denial. They see other people as the problem, not addiction, so they are hard to treat," Dean says.

Nurses in the addiction field are caring, but they tend to be tough. Failure is the hardest part of this job. There are clients who aren't going to make it and that is disheartening for nurses. It's difficult to see people they have worked so hard with relapse, but that is part of the reality of addiction. With many clients, nurses have to be aggressive and confrontational, and that brash style tends to carry over into work relationships. As a result, there is a lot of butting of heads, between doctors and nurses, and among nurses. "Because you have to be perceptive, and because you are always doing assessments, you tend to also be very demanding and critical of co-workers. We're really hard on each other," Dean says.

A particularly traumatic part of Dean's job is dealing with health professionals who are admitted for treatment. Addiction to drugs, and to prescription drugs in particular, is such a widespread problem that Homewood has a program specifically for doctors and nurses. "It's quite disturbing when you see people with the education and the knowledge and they still have a serious addiction. It shows you just how powerful it can be," Dean says.

Many nurses are superb caregivers because they have obsessive-type personalities, but the dark side of that personality trait is that they take their jobs home with them. Because of the stress and the isolation—much of it brought about by cutbacks and shift work—they turn to alcohol and sleeping pills. The tragic irony is how little support health-care institutions provide to their workers and, as a result, just how bad problems become before help is sought.

Dean, a long-time psychiatric nurse, has not had an addiction problem herself, but working in the field has dramatically changed her view of the profession. She moved to Homewood as a casual worker after being laid off from a full-time job. The downgrading was involuntary, but it ended up being a blessing in disguise. "At first part-time was not a choice, it was what I could get. But I realized that I was working really hard full-time and I was missing my life. Nursing can be an all-consuming job if you let it. That's why there's such a high burnout rate. Now I enjoy my work more, and I enjoy my life more," she says.

The Pink Room—Fred Haines

It's early evening, and a well-dressed, middle-age man walks into Emergency at Royal University Hospital in Saskatoon. He tells the triage nurse about a nagging pain in his stomach, and says that he would like to see a doctor. When she probes for details, the man replies that things haven't been going too well at work, that he's been a bit down and having these thoughts ...

The nurse tells the man to have a seat, someone will be right with him. She casts a glance just across the hall to the office of Fred Haines. He walks over, takes the file, and invites the man to come with him where they can talk privately.

The scene repeats itself several times throughout the evening, with manic teenagers, young mothers with post-partum depression, and street people. Police will come in with a babbling university student, or parents with a seemingly hyperactive child.

About one in every twenty people who go to hospital emergency rooms has mental-health problems, not physical ones. "The stereotype of the foaming-at-the-mouth, screaming lunatic is not accurate at all. I see people from all walks of life. If there is a trait most of them have in common it is that they are young and scared," says Haines, an emergency-intake-liaison nurse. Typically, patients range in age from 18 to 30, though preteens are increasingly joining the ranks of the mentally ill.

Because most nurses in Emergency do not like dealing with mental illness, or they are not equipped to do so, the majority of emergency rooms in urban centres now have at least one psychiatric nurse on staff. Even in a relatively small city such as Saskatoon, this trend towards specialization is both practical and cost-effective. Deciphering the musings of a schizophrenic who is not taking his medication is far more difficult than dealing with stab wounds or a burst appendix. And because many psychiatric patients are not forthcoming about what really ails them—masking the problem behind physical pains—and want, more than anything else, to vent, they require a lot of time.

In his first months on the job, Haines found that patients who routinely took three or four hours of staff time could be dealt with in an hour by a psychiatric nurse. They could also be seen a lot faster, after only thirty-seven minutes' wait on average. "Traditionally, psych patients have always been placed at the bottom of the list—after trauma, after major medical, after minor medical. In many emergency rooms, mental-health issues get dealt with only after the coughs and colds," Haines says.

Unfortunately, the cases that are truly emergencies, the acutely depressed and suicidal, are those that tend to get short shrift. "The florid psychotic is easy to spot, and easy to deal with. The people I really need to see are the quiet and withdrawn ones who will sit in the corner for six hours without saying anything. They are well kept, well nourished, and look to be in good health, but are really at risk. If they fall through the cracks, they could easily end up dead," he says.

Alongside the examination rooms in Emergency is the Pink Room. Instead of the exam table, sink, and sundry pieces of medical equipment, it has a couch and chairs. The name comes from the fact that it is painted entirely pink, supposedly a soothing colour. Haines dismisses the common belief that his patients are violent. Unlike most emergency-room nurses, who deal with a lot of violent drunks, he has never been hit. Unlike other nurses, he does not wear a uniform, but casual clothes, again to put people at ease. He is also slight and soft-spoken, which he says helps.

When a patient is deemed to have a mental-health problem— and while most self-refer, they can come in as failed suicides, on a warrant, or be assigned by the triage nurse or shuffled over by a doctor after a physical exam—he or she sees Haines in the Pink Room.

The nurse fills out the paperwork, but his principal goal is to get people to open up. "I talk to them, concentrating on the here and now, on why they have really come to Emergency." He does not delve much into their history, because experience has revealed that one of things mental-health patients hate the most is having to repeat their entire medical history time and time again.

Research has shown that most people who come to Emergency already have a well-established therapeutic relationship with a counsellor, psychologist, or psychiatrist. "There are some new diagnoses, particularly among teenagers who are bipolar [manic depressive] or schizophrenic, but usually they come to us because of an acute exacerbation of a previously diagnosed illness," Haines says. It is the same way a cardiac patient would use Emergency if he had chest pains, or an asthmatic who had breathing problems.

A lot of psychiatric patients are, in the jargon of the workplace, "frequent flyers"—those who are recognized by ER nurses as regular and bothersome visitors. Haines says that, although these patients are treated with disdain, they tend to use his services efficiently; they are often struggling with a number of problems at once (drug abuse and disease at once as mental illness) and need modifications in their medication, or someone to talk to.

"If you're living in a rooming house and collecting welfare, it can be an ordeal to get an appointment with a mental-health professional, so it's easier to show up at Emergency and talk to the nurse. Some of the frequent flyers even call ahead to make sure I'm not too busy," he says.

Once Haines has done an initial interview, which takes between fifteen minutes and an hour, he analyses the case and presents it to a doctor (usually a psychiatric resident), along with a recommendation. Most of the time, the physician accepts the suggested plan of action and writes the appropriate prescription or admission. The nurse then has a follow-up meeting with the patient, giving him or her the prescription and a referral to a community agency (only rarely are patients admitted to a psychiatric bed for observation).

Haines's work day stretches from 3:30 P.M. to midnight, five days a week, hours determined by a statistical analysis of when mental-health patients visit Emergency. He believes there is a need for another shift overnight—nurses report an influx of psych cases during the "Witching Hour," 3:00 to 4:00 A.M.—and on weekends, but the funding is not available. He will usually see four to six patients in a night. Yet, like most nurses working in institutions, he has a lot more paperwork to complete than he has down time. Because most of his workday occurs when the offices of community groups and medical professionals he refers to are closed, a lot of referrals are done by fax and voicemail.

Psychiatry is, says Haines, making an analogy to the Cinderella story, "the ugly sister of Emergency. It's not the high-profile stuff that makes the front page of the newspaper, so it's not a priority for spending." It is the antithesis of emergency medicine; in this area of nursing, success is measured in tiny steps, not by bringing people back from the dead.

"In my business, we don't have the wonderful fanfare of trumpets and the declaration from on high of 'cured' or 'saved.' Down the hall they get that, particularly with the trauma patients," Haines says. "My clients go back into the community and they still have serious problems. And, yes, I am likely to see them again, but that's not an indication of failure. What we aim for is not a miracle cure, it's to have them lead a reasonably good life, and they can do that with appropriate supports. I comfort myself knowing that I do a small part to help rebuild lives," Haines says.

Part Six
THE NOT-SO-
GOLDEN YEARS

A World Too Wide

Together, cardiovascular disease, cancer, and respiratory disease account for the vast majority of cases of illness and death—and, by extension, health-care costs—in Canadians over the age of 45.

Despite a steady decline since 1970, heart disease is still the leading killer, accounting for 37 per cent of all deaths. Cancer in all its forms is a close second, with lung cancer leading the way. But there is hope. Detection rates are up, particularly for prostate and breast cancer, and, overall, mortality has been declining for more than twenty years.

Practically speaking, this means that in real life people do not, as they do in TV movies, drop dead from heart attacks or discover that they have terminal cancer and mere days to live. Rather, these diseases are increasingly detected earlier and require long-term, specialized care, much of it provided by nurses.

In Part Six, you will meet Denise Cassan, a busy cardiac nurse. She works in preadmission, prepping patients for surgery, a job that on the surface seems straightforward, but is not. It is just one example of how nursing is changing dramatically: Cassan's patients used to be in hospital for long stays, but now many have day surgery, putting a far greater onus on nurses to provide education and counselling, often within a restrictive time frame.

Cancer nurses must provide similar services. The agency Interlink Community Care Nurses was born out of necessity, created by nurses who saw a shocking void in the care of cancer patients, as a result of a combination of cutbacks and technological advances. As an oncology nurse entering the twenty-first century, Beth Pelton realizes that the disease itself is often the least of the worries of cancer patients. Like many people with chronic illnesses, cancer patients have reasonable access to state-of-the-art medical treatment but often fail when they try to tap into programs that will help them maintain a semblance of a normal life during treatment—even obvious things like babysitting, accessible housing, and medication.

Ideally, in a country that believes in publicly funded health care, the medical and social-service systems would be seamlessly interwoven, but, in reality, they are far from it. Nurses all over the country work at breaking down those walls in the name of better patient care.

Darlene Orr, for example, serves that function at one of the lodges in a network operated by the Canadian Cancer Society. With increased specialization and regionalization, many cancer patients now have to travel far from their homes to get cancer treatment. The cancer lodges provide low-cost room and board to those undergoing chemotherapy and radiotherapy, as well as a supportive environment. Nurses also ensure that patients return home with the necessary supports, such as home care and homemaking.

In fact, home care is one of the fastest growing areas of nursing. More than 20,000 nurses nationwide now make house calls. Contrary to popular belief, this service is not primarily for the frail elderly (who tend to require homemaking services such as cleaning and shopping, more than they need home medical help). Rather, health boards and hospitals are moving care such as intravenous-drug treatments, wound management, and chronic-disease management into the community.

Janice Cibart is a home-care nurse in Regina whose clientele consists primarily of people with diabetes. About 3 per cent of Canadian adults have diabetes; it is a disease with socio-economic underpinnings. Poor people are far more likely to have diabetes, including one in every ten seniors and almost one in five aboriginal people. Cibart's home visits are important not only for the health of individual patients, but for the financial health of the health-care system. Studies showed that many of her clientele, because they cannot afford transport or feel uncomfortable in the traditional health-care setting, would skip their appointments. Poorly managed, diabetes can lead to serious heart disease, and significant expenses to both the health and social-welfare systems, so getting a nurse out in the community pays dividends quickly.

Regardless of how well people take care of themselves, they still fall ill and sometimes require surgery, which, of course, still takes place in hospitals. More than 1.1 million Canadians undergo surgical procedures each year. Three-quarters of all surgeries performed fall into five broad categories: obstetrical, 33 per cent; digestive system, 13 per cent; reproductive organs, 10 per cent; musculoskeletal, 10 per cent; and cardiovascular, 5 per cent. One of the most dramatic developments in medicine in the past generation has been the improvements in surgery, specifically the ability to perform transplants.

Janet Bate is a Halifax nurse who works in that highly specialized field. There are only about 1,500 organ transplants performed in Canada each year, and the veteran nurse participates in almost one hundred of them, putting her at the forefront of her profession. What troubles Bate, however, is the number of people waiting for organs. There are more than 3,000 Canadians on waiting lists, most of them hoping for kidneys. This is an example of the unfulfilled potential of nurses. Where there is a coordinated organ-retrieval system—usually overseen by a nurse—donation rates tend to skyrocket.

Studies show that transplant recipients live an average of ten years longer than those who continue on dialysis, their quality of life is much improved, and they save the public health system a bundle. Five years of follow-up treatment after a kidney transplant costs about $50,000; on the other hand, five years of dialysis costs about $250,000. In other words, for every 100 transplants, for every 100 kidneys retrieved, the health system will save $20 million.

Most of the savings achieved in the health system of late have not been of this variety. Rather, administrators opted for "savings" that came from laying off tens of thousands of nurses, an approach that has proved short-sighted and counter-productive, and has prompted much public dissatisfaction.

As baby boomers age, they are forcing the health system to become more consumer-oriented. Being on the front lines, and often serving in the role of consumer advocates, nurses have been the first to hear and respond to these demands. And many of them, frustrated at the conservatism of the public system, are turning to private enterprise to pursue their interests in areas such as health promotion. Mary Neill is a pioneer in a field that has tremendous growth potential and a broad range of opportunities for nurses. She left a secure but frustrating hospital job to found The Welcare Centre, a private clinic that focuses on people who, rather than sit back and let sickness catch up with them, want to take control of their health and wellness—in large part, menopausal women.

Today, not only are nurses opening new avenues of practice for themselves, but hiring has begun anew in the public-health system. For the sake of consumers and nurses alike, one hopes that it will be done with more foresight and wisdom than the layoffs, allowing nurses to promote wellness in addition to providing illness care, an approach that will produce real savings over time.

You Gotta Have Heart—Denise Cassan

Nursing has changed a lot in recent years, but nowhere more than in surgery. The combination of technological advances and fiscal restraints means that same-day admissions are becoming the norm, even in complex cases such as heart surgery, and patients are often discharged within hours of awaking from anaesthetic. Policies to delay admission and speed discharge place stress not only on patients and doctors, but on nurses, who see their ability to care and prepare put under severe time constraints.

As a nurse in the same-day admission unit of the Ottawa Heart

Institute, Denise Cassan knows these pressures well. At 6:00 A.M., she and a colleague greet six patients who will go under the knife within two hours of arriving at the hospital. Half of them will have heart surgery such as a bypass, while the other three will undergo angioplasty, a technique in which a balloon is inflated inside a vein or artery to flatten plaque (mostly cholesterol and lipids) that accumulates and leads to arteriosclerosis (hardening of the arteries).

All the patients have had some cardiac event but are getting treatment, so the surgery is considered elective. With waiting lists stretching to six months and beyond, however, many of them have been awaiting the day for a long time. "They're pretty tense and nervous when they arrive, so one of the first things we have to do is get them to relax," says Cassan.

The prep nurse has to get the patient undressed and shaved and answer all the questions—and there can be many, despite her education work in the weeks leading up to the day. Although heart surgery is now fairly routine, most patients want to spend a little time alone with close family members. They then get a visit from the anaesthetist and are given oxygen, and then are wheeled off to the operating room by the nurse. "It's pretty well one-on-one care, but the window's pretty tight. We don't have any time to sit around," says Cassan. While she is aware that many hospitals are trying to replace nurses and have technicians and orderlies do much of this preparation, she balks at the idea. "I guess you could have technicians do blood work, shaving, et cetera, but you would need several so you wouldn't save money. The thing about a nurse is that she can do it all, plus she can interpret the results," she points out.

At 12:30 P.M., another group of patients arrives to be prepped for surgery at 3:00 P.M., and the routine is repeated. Unless, of course, something has gone wrong. If a doctor is late or there is a long wait for an anaesthetist (a field where there are chronic shortages), the whole schedule can be thrown off. And if there is an emergency surgery—not at all uncommon in the cardiac field—one or more of the elective patients will get bumped. "And guess who has to deal with that? The nurse," Cassan says. "There is a lot of build-up to these operations, and when we have to tell people at the last minute that it's been cancelled, they're not usually too happy."

On a good day, between the two batches of admissions, the nurses prepare for the coming days, with lots of phone calls and patient visits. If time permits, Cassan will drop in on patients in post-op (where she worked for five years) because she knows how reassuring it is for them to see a familiar face when they wake up.

Ottawa Heart Institute is a world-class institution, renowned for its surgical expertise and nursing care. The cutbacks have not hit there as much as at some other hospitals. Still, the preadmission unit was operating on a ward that was shut down, and was moved to a clinic space. "Now our space is terrible, it's really inappropriate. But the people who make these decisions don't seem to think about practical issues like the lack of beds," Cassan says.

Hospital cuts have created bitterness and division among nurses. Cassan says the hardest part of her job is the ribbing that comes from other nurses. "Some of the other nurses, the ones on the ward, say: 'Two or three patients, that's the life.' They think it's a cushy job. But they don't realize the time constraints, that everything has to function like clockwork. It's not a cushy nursing job, it's just a different kind of work, and some people resent that," she points out.

Like many nurses today, Cassan is a part-time worker who, because of shortages, works full-time hours. Even her holidays are strictly controlled. The clinic closes for three weeks each summer, and that is her time off—without pay. But after fifteen years as a floater, she appreciates the regularity of day shifts, something she says will prolong her career by several years. "I was seriously thinking of retirement because I couldn't handle the shifts anymore," she says.

The day-surgery shift starts at 6:00 A.M. and wraps up at 2:00 P.M. Cassan also works in the preadmission unit, a shift that runs from 8:30 A.M. to 4:30 P.M. In that job, she has to make sure patients are suitable for same-day surgery and that they will be ready when they come in for their operation.

The initial visit, which usually comes after a referral from a cardiologist and some history of heart disease, lasts about four hours. The first person the patient sees is Cassan, who will spend about an hour doing a physical examination, blood work, and detailed medical history, with particular emphasis on heart problems and medications. The patient then goes off for an electrocardiogram and X-rays while the nurse prepares the file, with appropriate highlights, for the physicians. Next, the patient will meet briefly with a surgeon, cardiologist, and anaesthetist, who explain the procedure. Then it is Cassan's turn again, as she takes time to answer questions and do some education about pain control, intubation, and ventilator use (routine matters in cardiology) with the patient and family members. The nurse used to conduct a pre-op class as well, but now the hospital sends patients home with a video primer (one that was prepared by nurses).

In preadmission, Cassan will see between two and four patients per shift. The time between appointments is required to get lab results from others, do follow-up with doctors, and plan for coming visits. Most of the patients are men in their fifties and sixties, but the number of women with heart disease is growing steadily. Cassan says they "tend to be textbook cases: they have high cholesterol, smoke, and don't exercise. Most have some major lifestyle changes to make."

While the time to do education in the pre-surgery period is limited, she says many patients are hyper-aware and willing to learn, usually because they have been scared half to death by a heart attack and the realization that surgery is serious business. "A lot of heart patients change their lives dramatically in a short period, and that's uplifting to see as a nurse. Then there are the others—but they're really a minority—who come in with the pack of cigarettes tucked in their pocket, thinking surgery is a cure. That's frustrating to see."

Cassan says working in the cardiac field is rewarding because people are so appreciative that they have been given a second chance that they really have a zest for life before and after surgery. Some of that enthusiasm has rubbed off on her over the years, and she has become increasingly involved in community work.

Cassan is active on the health-promotion committee of the Heart and Stroke Foundation, and regularly volunteers to conduct blood-pressure clinics at the local shoping malls and in work-places. She is on the local committee of the Canadian Council of Cardiovascular Nurses, teaches cardiopulmonary resuscitation (CPR) both in the hospital (doing recertification for other nurses) and in the community, and has been involved with St. John Ambulance for many years.

But Cassan gives most of her hours to fundraising for the Ottawa Heart Institute itself. For many years, she has been one of the on-air volunteers for its annual fundraising telethon and, in 1999, graduated to co-hosting the event, which raised $2.6 million. She also participates in the hospital's other fundraising activities, such as the Manotick Fun Walk, a walkathon that features successful cardiac-surgery patients. It is this type of commitment that has earned the cardiac nurse "employee of the year" honours and many letters of thanks from former patients.

But Cassan downplays her achievements, saying that, like many nurses, she does not stop being a nurse, a caregiver, when she leaves her shift at the hospital. "Heart disease affects so many people and their families that you just get drawn in. Working at the hospital getting them ready for surgery is not enough. I feel I should get involved in the community too, doing prevention work. It's just another way of using my skills, and hopefully it makes a difference."

Support Is Somebody's Job — Beth Pelton

According to *Barron's Medical Dictionary*, cancer is an "abnormal, malignant growth of cells that invade nearby tissues and often spread to other sites in the body, interfering with the normal function of affected sites." The definition barely scrapes the surface, because cancer can also gnaw at your soul, deplete your savings, wipe out your job prospects, and tear apart your family.

Oncology nurses can treat the physical symptoms, but patients are often left to fend for themselves against the financial, social, and emotional repercussions of the overwhelming diagnosis. Interlink Community Care Nurses, a Toronto-based non-profit agency, was created to fill that void.

"The health-care system is becoming more specialized than ever and an unfortunate result is that people are being lost in the system more than ever," says Beth Pelton, a veteran Interlink nurse. "Most people come to an oncologist's office with a lot of other issues, and they can't keep the cancer piece separate. In fact, cancer is often a very small problem next to the other stuff. It's not humane to say 'Sorry, that other stuff is not my job.' It has to be somebody's job."

For an increasing number of patients, that somebody is family and friends. But, when they can't cope, or when the person is alone, Interlink is there. It was founded in 1987* by two oncology nurses who were frustrated by the fact that support services existed in the community but many of their patients did not have the knowledge or the energy to access them. Today, hundreds of Ontario cancer patients—many of them single, poor, and elderly, a demographic slice where the killer disease is increasingly prevalent—have nurses doing that work for them, and the agency is hoping to go national.

"Never mind chemotherapy, a lot of my job is accessing financial resources to get them through the day," Pelton says. She does not provide hands-on medical care (though she is qualified to do so), but rather advocacy and support.

If a patient does not know how to access home-care services, or has inadequate help, Pelton will approach the local Community Care Access Centre. A person with cancer may need social housing,

---

* The launch was made possible by a $1-million founding grant from the Atkinson Charitable Foundation.

social assistance, or help getting to the food bank. Because of the devastating effects of the disease, a patient may need babysitting to get some rest, or her children may need tutoring. Cancer may be the last straw in an already frayed marriage, and counselling may be as important as chemo. The patient may be too exhausted to do chores and may need a volunteer to shovel the walk, or help with an income-tax return complicated by medical expenses. None of that comes with the oncologist's prescriptions.

A distinguishing feature of Interlink is that it is the only program in the country where patients have direct access to nursing care; the only eligibility criterion is a cancer diagnosis. Further, the agency guarantees that it will respond to every inquiry within forty-eight hours, and service is free. (Interlink gets funding from Cancer Care Ontario, the provincial agency that oversees treatment in the province, and does private fundraising, but charges no fees.)

Each nurse has a caseload of about sixty patients at a time. Pelton will make three or four home visits daily (by contrast, many home-care nurses will now make a dozen), and a number of phone calls. "The beauty of independent practice is that nobody tells me that the patient has been allocated only half an hour. I take the time I need," she says.

During an initial visit, the nurse will usually just listen to patients' stories. Patients can range from newly diagnosed cases who have yet to see an oncologist through to quite advanced, even palliative, patients. "Above all, they appreciate a visit from someone who can just listen. No matter how catastrophic things seem, feedback often puts people at ease; it makes them feel less alone and more in control," Pelton says.

At the beginning, she will often educate, explaining in detail how their particular form of cancer progresses, and explaining chemotherapy/radiotherapy and the side effects it will cause. Then the questions come. Pelton says that Canada has a highly developed health-and-social-welfare system, but that it is not very consumer-friendly, particularly for people hit suddenly by a catastrophic illness such as cancer. An Interlink nurse acts as broker, wading through the complexity and pointing people in the right direction.

Pelton says patients often have very modest requests—Can they get transportation home from chemo, because they are afraid they might throw up in public? Can someone tell a child's school-teacher why he is distracted? What can you tell me about this experimental drug I read about on the Internet?—but they really do not have any clue where else to get answers. The sleuthing is sometimes difficult, particularly when a nurse gets enmeshed in the social-welfare bureaucracy, but, after years on the job, Pelton has developed a rich network of contacts that leaves her convinced she can solve almost any problem. "Every one of us at Interlink has a motto: 'There's gotta be something out there and we're gonna find it for you,'" she says.

The only request that repeatedly stumps her is: "Tell me I'm going to be all right." Unfortunately, in many cases, she cannot. More than half of all adult cancer patients will die, often in the short term. What advances in medicine have done is prolong life with the disease, often a mixed blessing. Interlink provides assistance with pain management both directly—the nurses all have at least five years experience in oncology—and by referral. There are volunteer groups such as Healing Touch Canada and Therapeutic Touch Canada that are popular with people with cancer. When treatments have been exhausted, Pelton can also help patients choose the palliative care they want. (Most people with terminal illnesses now choose to die at home, usually with a nurse at their side.)

Interlink's philosophy is to respect the patient's wishes. If someone decides to refuse chemotherapy in favour of a macrobiotic diet, Pelton will help find a store that sells macrobiotic foods and a dietician to offer advice. Similarly, she will track down suppliers of herbal medicine for those who eschew Western treatments. "What cements the relationship between the patient and the nurse, what makes it very special, is that they know we are there exclusively for them. We will support their decisions 100 per cent," Pelton says.

As Interlink becomes better known, it gets an increasing number of calls from other health professionals. Home-care nurses will call for advice on treating patients with cancer, as will family physicians. Oncologists now routinely make referrals, as does the Canadian Cancer Society. Pelton will also get involved on the medical side, if she deems it necessary. For example, when one of her clients began vomiting spontaneously, experience told her it was not a side effect from drugs but a brain lesion linked to her breast cancer; in that case, the nurse ensured that the woman saw her oncologist immediately. "Sometimes, I'm in a home and I start making calls and, after a while, the patient says: 'Oh my goodness, I just couldn't do this. I would just give up.' Cancer patients just don't have the energy to do everything required," Pelton explains.

But what about the many thousands of cancer patients who don't have the services of Interlink? Pelton believes people die a lot sooner, and that their quality of life is much diminished. A year's worth of service from an Interlink nurse costs about the same as a single day in hospital, so it doesn't take long for the nurse to pay dividends. The concept, obviously, could also be carried over to illnesses other than cancer. After all, people with chronic lung disease, Parkinson's disease, or Alzheimer's need just as much help muddling through the system.

Right now, Interlink is caught in a catch-22: it draws effusive praise but it is told it's too small, that it doesn't help enough people. Yet, governments will not step forward with money to help it expand and broaden its target audience. The initial concept for Interlink was to build a series of offices across the country where sick people could go to nurses for help, but governments did not buy into the idea. "I think the system has trouble dealing with supportive care, the stuff that nurses do best. It only understands medical care, but that's a tiny part of what patients need," Pelton says. But her most convincing argument for expansion is a devastatingly understated critique of the entire health and welfare system. Cold and alienating, it needs an infusion of caring, Pelton says. "If everyone in the system did their job 100 per cent of the time, we wouldn't need Interlink nurses. But they *are* needed—more than ever."

Nurse, Food, Lodging—Darlene Orr

At first blush, the words "cancer lodge" seem like an oxymoron. But the receptionist is chipper and, at midafternoon, the lounge behind her is bustling with activity: a foursome—two of them in pyjamas—playing bridge; a tiny girl in her Sunday best squealing with delight as Grandpa surprises her with candy; a bald 20-year-old flopped in front of the TV watching soaps; and a whistling volunteer rushing in to help a neatly coiffed older woman with a walker get to her appointment on time.

"Oh, the lodge is not a sad place to be at all," supervisor Darlene Orr says as she begins a tour of the Vancouver Island Lodge of the Canadian Cancer Society in Victoria. "People with cancer are normal here, and that's important. You can just be yourself without any of the stigma."

Because of specialization and regionalization trends across the country, many patients have to travel farther for cancer treatment, and lodges have become essential. While some hospitals in smaller centres offer basic chemotherapy, everyone on Vancouver Island who needs radiotherapy or more advanced chemotherapy now travels to Royal Jubilee Hospital for treatments. Most people with cancer are now treated as out-patients; since they do not get a hospital bed, they need a place to stay during treatment, which can vary from a few days to six weeks.

As a result, charitable groups such as the Canadian Cancer Society have stepped in to create networks of moderately priced hostels and lodges to ease the burden on individuals. The Victoria facility, plain but comfortable, costs $30 a night for accommodation and meals, substantially less than a hotel. And, unlike hotels (and many lodges, for that matter), it is staffed around the clock by a nurse. "We're responsible for everything from making sure patients are comfortable, pain-wise, to maintenance of the building," Orr says. She also collects research data, does accounting, and links patients up to services in their communities, such as home care. "It's like being a house mother with a medical bag on one arm," she says.

The focus of the nurse's work is symptom management, helping people deal with the pain, nausea, grief, and the many losses that come with the disease. For a lot of people, the period between diagnosis and treatment is just a whirlwind, so, when they get to the lodge and settle in, the cancer diagnosis really hits them. They can be quite emotional.

Yet, it is not the kind of place where people sit in their rooms crying, or where they will be found huddled sick in a corner. Rather, they reach out to each other and to the volunteers—many of them cancer survivors—for support, and the nurse acts as a combination caregiver and facilitator. "I don't do as much for them as they do for themselves; I do the linking. But I know it works because they're always looking out for each other, laughing and playing practical jokes," Orr says.

For nurses one of the attractions is that they get to know patients and their families intimately, and often build lasting bonds. (Orr says nurses maintain correspondence with many of their charges for years after they go home.) "The challenge in this job is to see past the disease to the person, but when you do it's so rewarding," she says. The disease, however, cannot help but make an impact, and the nurses tend to be active Cancer Society volunteers, canvassing and participating in other fundraising events.

Patients staying at the lodge range in age from 16 to 99, but the average is just over 65. Lung cancer is the most prevalent, followed by throat, prostate, and breast cancer, but patients often have ailments other than cancer itself. The average stay is seven days. To be eligible for admission, patients have to be able to care for the majority of their personal needs. About one in three brings family members along to help, but the nurse will assist some residents with eating, bathing, and getting to the cancer clinic. At any given time, about half the residents will be doing fine, and that's the only way a single nurse can handle a patient load of twenty-nine. But for those suffering side effects of treatment and emotional distress, Orr plays an important role in administering pain medication, changing dressings, and, above all, being available when they want to talk.

At a time when some lodges for cancer patients and others with severe medical conditions are doing away with nurses to save money, Orr is adamant that they are essential. "If you provide just beds and meals, why bother? You would miss out on physical and emotional support, and that's what counts. Many lodges will want to wrap my knuckles for saying this, but they're being short-sighted, they're letting the budget take priority over the patient, and that's not right."

While the medical response to cancer gets most of the attention and funding, Orr notes that a radiation treatment takes about fifteen minutes. Patients who are far away from home and alone spend most of the other twenty-three hours and forty-five minutes of their day at the lodge, and that time is obviously going to have an impact on their medical outcome. "You can feel lousy and I can let you cry, maybe even cry myself, and I feel there is some achievement in that, I feel that is an important part of care," the nurse says. "I will not change the fact whether the patients live or die, but I will change how they cope. I will give them some control, and I think that's often critical to their well-being, physically and emotionally."

Because the facility is resident-oriented, there is not a lot of structure. Asked how a typical day unfolds, Orr just chuckles, and reaches for her agenda book. "Okay, today's pretty typical. I started with a report, helped someone get breakfast; I checked on a couple that was having a little trouble, and had a chat; I came downstairs to get a taxi for a patient, then met with some volunteers; I snuck into the office for a bit to work on a report for head office." She pauses to answer another question from someone who has popped her head in the door. "Then, I left to check on a patient who went to Emerg yesterday; did a little follow-up with family back in their community; I assisted a person who was unable to eat alone; took someone to the clinic because the volunteers were swamped; I found an electrician because the cooler is broken; I did a tour for someone scheduled for radiation; took a booking for next week; talked to a student with a cancer-related project; that takes us almost to noon. ... I would like to say it's a fun job, but that would make it sound frivolous."

As a nurse, however, Orr is in an enviable position. There is no shift work. The job is not very physically demanding. She does not report to a physician or a nursing body. Her employer, the Canadian Cancer Society, allows her great autonomy, insisting only that she balance the budget and always put the interests of patients first. "In a hospital, you are often left with the impression that patients are in the way. Here, I can develop policies that make their lives better. I can institute change without going through a huge bureaucracy. When patient care needs to be improved, we do it, no questions asked. I don't think there's a single nurse in a hospital who can say the same thing," she points out.

For Orr, after two decades in the hospital setting, landing a job at the cancer lodge was a dream come true. She left a hospital management position to take—at a substantial pay cut—a casual position with the charitable organization, and has never regretted the move for a second.

"My stomach still ties in knots every time I walk into a hospital, just the memories of the stress. It's easier nursing here than in any hospital: there's no hierarchy and we're really open about our feelings. In a hospital, you have be tough. Here there's Kleenex on every table and we're never afraid to use them," Orr says.

Unlike many nurses, Orr is not planning on an early retirement. On the contrary: "People ask me if I'll stay in this job till I'm 65. Are you kidding? I'll be pushing my walker around here and still not want to retire. I wanted to be a nurse to make a difference in people's lives, and here I make a difference every single day."

Nurse in the 'Hood—Janice Cibart

Janice Cibart carves a parking spot out of the snowbank with her pickup, then trudges up the unshovelled walk. The door is open and she hollers "Hello" in lieu of knocking. Her client, a 61-year-old truck driver who had quadruple bypass surgery a couple of months earlier, is watching TV and, as a gesture of welcome, he hits the mute button. Cibart asks about his grandchildren, his horses, then, as she lays out her supplies on the foot rest, guides the conversation around to his diet and health.

"Bacon and eggs?" the nurse asks.

"Only a couple of times this week," he says, smiling and explaining to the visitor that, before his surgery, bacon and eggs were a staple, the meal of choice twice a day while he was on the road.

"Great. Just great," Cibart responds as she is peeling off a dressing covering a lingering leg wound, the result of poor circulation caused by his diabetes. Along with the wound care, she has been doing nutritional teaching and monitoring the patient's use of insulin and heart medication. He complains about "feeling funny" each time he takes one of the pills, so the nurse makes a couple of calls, to the pharmacist and the physician. She urges him to bring the matter up at the next doctor's appointment, scheduled for the next day, and asks if he needs a ride.

Cibart works as a home-care nurse for the Regina Health District. She is responsible for all the "complex aboriginal patients" in the city, though many live in a poor area in the northwest dubbed "The 'Hood." In a population that has one of the worst health outcomes—urban aboriginals—she is responsible for the ongoing care of forty to fifty of the toughest, chronic cases.

"The hard thing at the beginning was developing trust, to get people to let me in the door. They know now that I'm there to treat them, not to judge them, " Cibart says.

In a typical day, Cibart will see eight to ten patients. At one of her first calls, the patient, a blind diabetic woman who is getting treatment for foot ulcers, refuses to let the nurse in the house. She is drunk and angry. Cibart returns to her truck and makes a note to come back later in the week. Her attitude is that whatever goes on within the four walls of their houses is none of her business. This philosophy is a mainstay of community nursing.

At a later appointment, with a 38-year-old quadriplegic who needs his catheter irrigated, the issue of drug abuse comes up again. The patient tells her that he's marking an important milestone: six months without injection drugs (though he is taking various other drugs orally). Cibart is supportive and encouraging. "I like to spend a little extra time with him because he's doing so well. He couldn't get a ride to the clinic for methadone, so he kicked the habit all alone," she says. The patient has also educated her. "When I started the job, I was really naïve about drugs. He's taught me a lot of stuff, really practical stuff that helps me do my job. Say, somebody is abusing Lysol, or sniffing glue; that can really throw their diabetes out of whack," she says.

More than 1.5 million Canadians have diabetes.* A manageable disease, it is nonetheless the leading cause of blindness, kidney failure, and amputation. A disease whose symptoms snowball, it is also a major cause of high blood pressure, heart disease, and stroke. It costs the Canadian health-care system an estimated $9 billion annually. In the aboriginal community, diabetes is an epidemic and, particularly among those who do not take their insulin or medication, it is the leading killer.

Much of Cibart's work consists of monitoring blood-sugar levels and preparing insulin syringes and oral medications to encourage severe diabetics to control their disease and thus avoid further complications. Yet, as she has learned over the years, diabetes is often well down the list of concerns for her clients. "If they cut off the power in the middle of the winter, one of your kids is in jail, you have no food in the fridge, and your cheque is late, then you're not going to spend a lot of time thinking about whether you took your needle that day," the nurse says.

---

* Type 1 diabetes occurs when the pancreas no longer produces insulin, a condition that strikes early in life. Treatment is a daily insulin injection. Type 2 diabetes usually appears after the age of 45. It occurs when the body can't effectively use the insulin produced by the pancreas, and can be treated with a combination of diet, exercise, and oral medication. About one in twenty pregnant women develops gestational diabetes, and almost half of them develop type 2 diabetes later in life.

Home care is essential in these cases because otherwise patients would get no treatment at all. People have no cars or money to get to clinics. Cibart points to one of her clients, a 48-year-old Métis woman who developed diabetes during pregnancy. She has since lost her vision, had a leg amputated, and receives regular dialysis due to kidney failure. "She hasn't been to the diabetes clinic for three years. She has other problems. As a non-treaty Indian, she has no drug benefits, no housing allowance; she's really struggling to survive."

As demanding as the job is, Cibart loves it because she is out in the community. There are always a lot of children around and, in many ways, she ends up treating whole families, not just a specific family member. "If the mother is compliant, if her diabetes is under control, that's going to have a huge impact on the whole family," she says. "And while I'm there I can talk to the kids about nutrition, about birth control, all kinds of stuff."

Before moving to home care, Cibart worked for fourteen years as a pediatric nurse, did stints as a nurse in a Nepalese women's prison, and spent another period in remote African villages treating women and children with HIV-AIDS. Many of the challenges she faced in Africa exist in Regina. While diabetes (and its offshoots) is the mainstay of her practice, Cibart treats a variety of conditions. She has a growing number of patients with HIV-AIDS, hepatitis, tuberculosis, and other conditions that stem from drug and alcohol abuse and poverty. "One of my patients is a pregnant IV-drug user who has HIV, hep B, hep C and a few other issues. That's the level of complexity I see pretty routinely," she says.

The most difficult part of the job, however, is grasping the social, not medical, complexity, of cases. She often has trouble getting other medical professionals to understand that reality. Cibart cites the example of a client who became a paraplegic after a car crash. He returned for follow-up surgery that included extensive skin grafting. The young man was supposed to remain in hospital, confined to bed, for eight weeks, but checked himself out after less than a week. After a couple of days, he called Cibart and asked for help.

"A lot of conventional medicine is not conducive to my clients' lifestyle. This guy is a heavy smoker and drinker and they tell him to stay in bed for eight weeks without access to cigarettes or alcohol. There's no way that's going to happen," she explains. In cases like that one, Cibart becomes an advocate. The plastic surgeon refused to see the client because he had left the hospital, so the nurse eventually got permission to remove the man's staples herself and continue follow-up treatment in the home.

A common practice in the aboriginal community is turning to traditional healers, which many mainstream doctors frown upon. "If people discontinue their insulin because they want to use traditional medicine, I don't judge them. My role is to treat them as best I can—according to their wishes," Cibart says.

Where home-care nurses tend to find support is from their colleagues. It is tough, isolating work, even in the best of circumstances, so they make a point of meeting informally. Every morning, a half-dozen nurses will gather at Butter Tart Bakery for a kaffeeklatsch. They know the job they do really saves the system money. They have clients who would otherwise never get treatment, whose condition would deteriorate until it was quite serious. Others think nothing of going to Emergency two or three times a week. Cibart believes far too many take their own health for granted and close their eyes to others in need in their communities.

"When people say my patients are spoiled because the nurse goes to their house, or that home care is really expensive, I just laugh. I know I'm making a difference every day—on a lot of levels."

Every Bit as Important—Janet Bate

When Janet Bate first visited an operating room, as a nursing student, she fainted at the sight of a woman undergoing a Caesarean section. Not an unusual response, but a notable one, given her ultimate career choice as a nurse in one of the country's busiest transplant programs.

Her unit at Queen Elizabeth II Health Sciences Centre in Halifax is responsible for urology, oral surgery, and some transplants (not heart or lungs). Bate participates in about seventy transplants annually, mostly kidneys, plus hundreds of other surgical procedures.

"In OR it's sterile, all you see is blood," she says, dismissing her queasiness with twenty-five years of hindsight. "It's a lot easier on the stomach than being a floor nurse. I soon realized that cleaning up after incontinents and vomit was a lot more difficult than a little blood. Besides, it's a lot less gory now than when I started."

In fact, working as a charge nurse, Bate probably finds her goriest job to be conflict management. In fields like transplant medicine which tend to attract perfectionists (or "thoroughbreds," in the hospital jargon), clashes are inevitable. But nurses such as Bate, no-nonsense and sharp-witted, act as referees. She is also responsible for scheduling and assigning the seventeen nurses on the unit, and all the headaches that entails in a time of shortages.

The charge nurse orders supplies and books about forty cases a day in five operating rooms. She must make sure surgeries are scheduled properly, that all disciplines are present, and that the room is readied for the next patient. But, administratively, Bate's biggest headache has been weathering an amalgamation, one that she opposed. Bringing together nurses and surgeons from two hospitals was stressful, but, in the end, "we were lucky, the staff blended well," she says.

In addition to her duties as charge nurse, Bate spends a lot of time in the operating room. She has some scheduled shifts, but most nights and weekends the nurse is on call. Because transplants depend a lot on accidents (which, in large proportion, occur on Friday and Saturday nights), Bate works about three weekends out of four, but does not complain about her gruelling schedule. "I'm not making a sacrifice, I'm being selfish. I just love it in OR. I never get bored," she says. In fact, there was a time when she volunteered to come in on call without pay just to get more experience.

In the operating room, there are two nurses, circulating and scrub. The circulating nurse sets up the room, receives the patient, and stays with him until the operation. "Every patient who goes to surgery is nervous. I find the way to relax them is to explain the procedure—that's reassuring—and to crack a few jokes," Bate says. During surgery, the circulating nurse takes care of all the fluids, drugs, and monitoring, as well as the related paperwork. She is also responsible for sponges—about eighty are used per operation, and she cannot afford to misplace one—counting sutures, and emptying the catheter bag. If there is heavy bleeding or unexpected complications, she will be very busy. If a surgeon decides a biopsy is needed, the circulating nurse is responsible for the kit. During a transplant, she will also monitor time and blood loss, which can often be critical.

The scrub nurse also spends some time with the patient, doing a final pre-op assessment and getting consent forms signed. She will also help the anaesthetist set up, administer oxygen, catheterize, shave the patient (if necessary, and it often is in urology cases), and make sure the patient is well positioned. The scrub nurse also assists in setting up the room, with particular emphasis on instruments. She will scrub, gown, and glove herself and the surgeon, and pass instruments during the operation.

"There's a lot more that goes into handing a surgeon a scalpel than there appears to the untrained eye. I hand him every instrument before he asks. I know every detail of the procedure, and I study to keep up with the latest techniques. That keeps the operation going smoothly. Administrators don't have a clue about this, they think we're like robots, but the surgeons really appreciate the difference a good OR nurse can make," Bate says. Every instrument is also meticulously counted and monitored. An efficient nurse can bring surgery time down from three hours to two, and in complex procedures like transplants that can make a significant difference. "The nurses can make or break a transplant, there's no doubt about it," Bate says.

After the operation, the circulating nurse stays with the patient until he is delivered to post-op. In some hospitals, transport is an orderly's job, but top-level institutions such as Queen E II insist on a nurse-to-nurse transfer. That is because a trained eye is essential for spotting post-operative complications, and it is important for patients to have a nurse present when they awake from anaesthetic because it can be a frightening experience.

The nurses usually have between fifteen and thirty minutes between operations. In an eight-hour shift, it is not unusual for a nurse to participate in three oral surgeries and seven urology cases. Transplants, often done on call, with as little as thirty minutes' notice, can take up to five hours just in the operating room.

Bate has a particular affinity for kidney transplants, for a very personal reason. As a child, her twin brother lost a kidney and her parents always told her that, should his other kidney fail, it would fall on her to make a life-saving organ donation. (It turns out, however, that she is not a match, because they are not identical twins.) "I think this knowledge I had, from a very young age, about the ability of transplants to save lives was an inspiration to me," Bate says. And it is particularly intriguing for a transplant nurse today because living donations of kidneys (often from siblings) are becoming commonplace. Much satisfaction comes, she says, from knowing that transplants make such a dramatic difference in people's lives.

During her time in OR, Bate has witnessed many other advances. More than 60 per cent of surgery is now endoscopic, mostly for kidney stones. A special instrument, often a laser, is inserted, either into an orifice or through a tiny incision, and the surgery is performed while being viewed on a video screen. During endoscopy, there is no scrub nurse. Bate says high-tech instruments, often seen as labour-saving, actually place extra demands on nurses. For example, she needed a dozen hours of training before participating in prostate surgery using a Yaglaser. That particular bit of machinery also requires nurses to wear a 15-kilogram lead apron, compounding the strain on the back that comes from long hours standing in OR.

But, in the hospitals of today, Bate complains, administrators are much more enamoured with the surroundings and the equipment than with experienced personnel. "You can operate in a barn if you have the right instruments and the right people. But the most beautiful facility in the world will be of no use if you don't have the right nurses and the right surgeon in the OR," she points out.

Because she rarely misses a kidney transplant, Bate has developed an impressive level of expertise. "More than one surgeon has said to me: 'You could probably put this kidney in pretty fast.' But I know my limits, and I know my job," she says. "They mean it as a compliment, but what I really hate is when I hear people say: 'She's a great nurse, she should have been a doctor.' I'm proud of being a good nurse. I don't see it as a hierarchy, but parallel professions. In the OR, I'm every bit as important as the surgeon."

Yet, her youngest daughter, as fascinated as her mother by medicine, has opted to go to medical school (hoping, ultimately, to be a surgeon) instead of to nursing school. "I'm happy with her decision. I can't very well say to her: 'Don't. Become a nurse.' That would be hypocritical. But I think if you've got the intelligence and the opportunity to be a surgeon, strive for that first. I want my daughters not only to have fulfilling careers, but to be financially independent, and nursing won't allow them to do that."

Bate says the pay scale for nurses, particularly experienced, specialized ones, is pathetic. She notes that, during the last decade, while she has been continually upgrading her education (largely at her own expense) and working in a field that is increasingly complex, nurses have not had a raise in Nova Scotia. "We took a 3 per cent rollback because they said there was a financial crisis, then we went seven years without a raise. And they wonder why there are shortages. They wonder why nurses go to the States."

With her résumé, Bate would have no trouble landing a better-paying job in a larger centre in Canada or the Unites States, but she has opted for the quality of life in Halifax, for a stable family life. Like many nurses, she can permit herself that luxury because there are two wage earners in the family. Her satisfaction comes not from the paycheque, but from the challenges that arise in the operating room.

Bate's latest goal is to qualify for First Assist, an innovation in the heart-surgery program. In the pilot project—which, so far, is a hit—nurses assume many of the duties of a surgical intern, including, notably, harvesting the patient's vein while the surgeon is working simultaneously on the chest. Under the First Assist protocol, nurses can suture, tie up vessels, and retract, greatly expanding their hands-on role in the operating room. "If you keep nurses wanting to be nurses, if you give them these new challenges—and be more reasonable about pay—the profession will stay healthy; it will be able to renew itself," Bate says.

She is troubled by the fact that so many of her colleagues are burned out and lacking enthusiasm for their profession. "In twenty-three years of nursing, there has not been a single day that I have not learned something. I'm not sure many people can say that about their jobs."

A Change of Life—Mary Neill

Mid-life is a stressful time. The kids are growing up, maybe even moving out and leaving the nest empty. Parents are getting older, probably needing your care. Your marriage may be falling apart or drifting along aimlessly. Single or divorced, you may start worrying about who will take care of you when your health fails. The career-track jobs may no longer interest you or, worse yet, you could find yourself abruptly out of work. The little aches and pains may start catching up with you. Then there are the more dramatic physical changes, often accompanied by psychological ones.

Yet, a woman at this crossroads who reaches out to the health-care system is, more likely than not, going to end up with a prescription for hormone-replacement therapy. "A few pills: That's the answer to menopause. Then we're supposed to pretend that the emotional and psychological needs simply don't exist," says Mary Neill, a women's-health nurse and director of The

Welcare Centre in Toronto. "It's no wonder there's a frustration out there that's palpable. That medical model is archaic."

Only 20 per cent of prescriptions for hormone-replacement therapy are actually filled, and only half of those are followed. Some women will try them but dislike the side effects or weight gain that accompanies the medication. Others will forgo the treatment because they have heard there are increased risks of breast cancer. Yet, without the treatment, they could have a higher risk of heart attack. Many menopausal women will feel unwell for years, often to the point of needing antidepressants. The lack of treatment is also reflected in the number of broken hips among older women suffering from osteoporosis related to hormonal imbalances. "The cost of not doing things differently, the cost of neglect, is enormous," Neill says.

Women coming to Welcare for help dealing with their "change of life" will get the different kind of care that Neill espouses, that she thinks all women are entitled to. A first-time visit to the clinic starts with a lifestyle assessment, conducted by a nurse. She will spend an hour or more looking at a woman's eating habits, exercise programs, sleep patterns, medical history, and discussing what changes the woman wants to make, and why. There is a component that includes a doctor's visit, and many women choose hormone-replacement therapy. But the rate of using the prescriptions is almost 100 per cent, because the nurse does follow-up and adjustments can be made to medication.

The nurse's principal role, however, is promoting wellness, and she does so by acting as a coach. She will establish a six- to ten-week program and set goals along with the patient. The nurse may do referrals to a health club, a chiropractor, or a nutritionist. With some patients, she goes shopping and teaches label reading. Many patients use the technique of journaling, and the nurse discusses concerns that arise in follow-up visits. "It's all about building a relationship. The patient takes much more responsibility for her health, but she knows the nurse is there when she has questions or needs help," Neill says.

When she was director of nursing at Women's College Hospital in Toronto, between 1990 and 1998, Neill was frustrated by the fact that this kind of preventive-health model was not the norm, that many people would get no help until their health degenerated to the point of needing emergency services. "A lot of what we were seeing in Emerg was people who were afraid; there was lots of self-abuse, mismanagement of medication, but they didn't have to be there if care was delivered differently," she says.

Neill was also at the centre of a political storm as the Ontario government, as part of its health-care restructuring, planned to merge Women's College Hospital with Sunnybrook Health Sciences Centre and, many people believed, destroy the former in the process. (The institutions have now been merged and the amalgamation goes by the name Sunnybrook and Women's College Health Sciences Centre.) "It was always the same thing, cuts being made on the backs of nurses and prevention falling by the wayside. All our energy was spent fighting and it wasn't paying off. I decided I really needed to get out of the rat race," she says. Neill had already made an abrupt career change at age 30: a long-time dancer with the Royal Winnipeg Ballet, she left to become a nurse, and rose quickly to one of the top hospital jobs. Now she decided to start over again.

The hospital was well known for its community-outreach initiatives, most of them nurse-centred. Neill had worked on a community-based training program that had nurses teach women (many of them menopausal) to take better care of themselves, a program that won a Commonwealth Secretariat Award for Innovation in the health-care field. Sadly, one of the projects that died on the drawing board when Women's was swallowed up was a plan to expand on the notion and open a number of satellite sites dedicated to women's health. Neill had drafted business plans, scouted out locations, and sold investors and health-care bureaucrats alike on the merits of community-based preventive medicine. The plug was pulled, but she didn't want to let the project die.

A doctor who was sold on the idea became her partner and they established such a clinic under private ownership. Welcare opened in January 1998. "My experience in a hospital set me up beautifully for managing. Where I was really lacking was marketing skills. In a hospital there's never a shortage of people coming through the door, but it's different in a clinic." Neill says that, at the beginning, she wasted a lot of money marketing ineffectively. But now, instead of spending on advertising, she does a lot more grass-roots networking to attract clients.

About three times a month, she delivers public lectures on women's health. And she spends a lot of time doing the rounds of health clubs, naturopaths, massage therapists, health-food stores, human resource managers, and other places people interested in managing their health go looking for answers. Today, most of the clinic's business comes through word-of-mouth, and it is doing well. Naturally, a lot of that clientele is at mid-life, going through a re-evaluation and adapting to changes wrought by menopause and andropause.

"Over the years, the onus on self-care has been forgotten. The health-care system focuses almost exclusively on disease treatment, and that is doing us all a great disservice," Neill says. "Canadians are, generally, quite articulate about health, and there comes a point in all our lives when we want to act on that knowledge. But when [people] try to act on their common sense instincts—which are to avoid getting sick—they keep hitting this wall."

Neill admits the move to the private sector was difficult because she is a firm believer in this country's public health-care system. "As a Canadian, I value universal health care and I fear its erosion and destruction. But, on the other hand, when you try to use the services of a hospital, you are often frustrated; nobody ever has the time to tell you things, to explain. There are changes that need to be made, there are gaps to be filled, and I'm afraid innovation is going to have to come from the private sector, from clinics like this one that challenge the status quo," she says. "Where I see the business opportunity is in value-added care, in providing long-term support that maximizes health and well-being. It's a shame that's not provided in our system right now, as a matter of course, but I don't see money rushing into prevention any time soon."

Neill says that, while she feels a certain discomfort in charging people for services at the clinic, they are, by and large, happy to pay. And, ultimately, she feels her work will save the system a lot of money. "What I don't like is this blanket accusation that I'm hurting the health-care system because I'm in private enterprise. I don't agree with that at all."

Part Seven
THE FINAL YEARS

Mere Oblivion?

The most profound socio-economic change in society today is the ageing of the population. There are, for the first time in history, more people over the age of 55 than under the age of 15. The two fastest-growing age groups are the over-75 and over-85 categories. And the seniors' population is expected to double in the next half-century.

Numbers like this make health economists blanch. Seniors are, by far, the biggest consumers of health-care services. People over 65 make up only 13 per cent of the population, but they account for almost half of all public spending on health care. If seniors already cost the system four times more than young people, the reasoning goes, the public-health system is on the fast track to bankruptcy.

Yet, this disaster scenario is based on a stereotype—that ageing is synonymous with poor health. The reality is that seniors are living longer, healthier, and wealthier lives than at any time in history. Most live independently, in their own homes or with family. More than 80 per cent of those over the age of 65, and almost as many over the age of 75, describe their health as good, very good, or excellent. The death rate has fallen by 25 per cent in a generation. More than half of seniors exercise regularly, a rate about the same as for 25-year-olds. And the biggest predictor of poor health, poverty, is down sharply, in large part due to federal income supplements. In 1980, more than one in three seniors lived below the poverty line; today, the figure is less than one in five. Average income is still only $20,451, and almost 700,000 of

Canada's 3.7 million seniors still live in poverty, however. That, more than anything else, will pose a burden to the health-care system in the immediate future.

One of the great fallacies that pervades our thinking about health care, the one driving the disaster scenarios, is that sickness and poor health are inevitable in older people, that the emphasis must be in treatment rather than prevention.

Sonja Lundström, a nurse who does health-promotion work with seniors, and others in the growing ranks of public-health nurses in the gerontology field have demonstrated that educating seniors can be as effective as educating children, that many of the most effective measures are the simplest. This is not surprising, considering that the greatest health hazard to older people is, as it is for children, falls. In Canada, falls kill more than 5,000 people over the age of 65 each year; for every death, there are dozens of injuries such as broken hips and concussions. The total bill for falls is almost $8 billion—$1 of every $10 spent on health care. Falls are also the leading cause of institutionalization; once a person loses mobility, she or he is far more likely to end up in a nursing home.

When Lundström carries out simple tasks, such as measuring to see if a walker is the proper height, teaching a person with blood-pressure problems how to stand slowly, and rearranging furniture in a senior's apartment to prevent falls, she is saving the system money at a rate that cost-cutting bureaucrats could only dream of achieving with their ill-planned layoffs. Those little gestures also dramatically improve the quality of life of individuals, allowing them to continue living in the community.

What older people fear most is not dying, but loss of autonomy, of control, of dignity. Helene Henrichsen deals with a clientele that is suffering principally from heart disease, many of them considered too sick even to have surgery. But they have taken charge of their health by opting for chelation therapy, a treatment that is one of many complementary therapies available today—a $3-billion market, and growing. Henrichsen, an intravenous-therapy nurse, is expanding the boundaries not only of health care, but of the profession, as one of the growing legion of nurse-entrepreneurs.

Roxanne MacLeod also works for a for-profit company, in one of the fastest-growing parts of the health-care system: home care. In the past decade, the number of hospital visits by seniors has fallen by 15 per cent, more sharply than among any other age category. In the process, they have become the biggest users of home-care services. (There is no denying, however, that home care has not kept pace, and much of the burden of care has been taken up by family members.) For example, one in every five women over the age of 75 now gets home-care services. But, overall, only about 550,000 Canadians receive home care, and it accounts for less than 4 per cent of health-care spending in Canada. Recent studies have also shown that one in nine people who need home care is not getting it because it is too costly, an indictment of our failure to keep the public-health system current and relevant.

The principal reason for mobility limitations—the most likely reason seniors will get home care—is arthritis in women and back problems in men. In both women and men, the second reason is dementia. Fortunately, a full range of medical and health services can now be delivered in the home. Many patients feel more comfortable there than in an institution, and providing care in the home can be significantly cheaper—about $8,000 a year less on average, according to research—even for people who require sophisticated apparatus such as ventilators and intensive nursing care. (A dozen hours of nursing care still costs about half as much as a hospital bed for a day, and the patient gets more individual attention.)

There are almost 200,000 people currently living in nursing homes. Some of them would undoubtedly be better cared for at home, in a good palliative-care program, but, for many sick elderly, institutional care is appropriate. Increasingly, patients entering nursing homes do so because their condition has deteriorated to the point where home care has become too burdensome and costly—in particular, those who have health crises that require frequent hospital visits.

Madeleine Shorthill, a nurse in a long-term-care hospital, will tell you that this aspect of gerontological nursing has a poor reputation, and inappropriately so. Caring for the frail elderly—those we used to call the bed-ridden—is indeed hard work, but important. When people have nothing left but their dignity, caring for them, and keeping that dignity intact, is an art.

Listening to Merial Forde, a nurse who works with veterans with Alzheimer's disease, speak lovingly of her patients allowed me to truly understand what caring means. Her soft touch on a man's hand, the gentle lilt of her voice, calming his demons, said more to me about the art of nursing than any number of textbooks ever could. Hers is a nursing specialty that cannot be taught; it must be learned through years at the bedside.

Nursing specialization begins in the labour and delivery room, and it extends to death. Palliative care and hospice care are among the fastest-growing areas of nursing. Hospice nurses such as Carolyn Adams of Royal Victoria Hospital cannot prevent critically ill patients from dying, but they can influence the quality of their death. That means a lot, especially to family members. When nurses talk of a "good death," that is what they mean. It is not preventing the inevitable, it is not performing miracles, it is bringing a small measure of comfort to patients, with painkillers or soothing words. It is knowing that your presence makes a difference.

Golden Veins—Sonja Lundström

In the health-care field, seniors don't get a lot of good press. They get stereotyped as old, crotchety, and no longer very useful. They are also labelled as a costly, and ever-costlier, burden on the public health-care system, filling up hospital beds and clogging emergency rooms with their aches and pains.

"Nonsense," Sonja Lundström says emphatically. "It is true that a lot of seniors end up inappropriately in hospital or Emergency, but the only reason that happens is that we leave them with no choice, we don't provide them with appropriate care."

Lundström, a public-health nurse on the seniors'-health-resource team of the Winnipeg Community Long-Term Care Authority, is determined to change that sad reality. Only one of a handful of projects of its kind, the team is setting out to do what the public health-care system has never done well: practise preventive medicine for a population that ranges from 65 to 105.

"We have a consumer society. We have this idea that we don't have to take care of things; we just use them and, when they're old, we throw them away. That attitude carries over to people, to seniors. We don't want to take responsibility; we want to buy a cure," Lundström says. "But the reality is that most injuries can be prevented, and most illnesses can be avoided, or at least well managed, regardless of age."

The health-resource-team concept was launched in Winnipeg in April 1999,* but with an eye to the future. Within a decade, the seniors' population in the city is expected to grow by one-third, and policy-makers are looking for ways to break this age group's costly dependency (albeit by default) on hospital care. Still in its infancy, the team has a specific target: 13,374 seniors who live in five high-density apartment blocks in northeast Winnipeg. The clientele is principally of Eastern European background, working class, and no-nonsense—in other words, a microcosm of much of Canada's ageing population. "In a few years, we're going to have data on effectiveness of this kind of intervention; we're going to know how much of a difference we can make," Lundström says.

The nurse plays a central role on the team. Along with an occupational therapist, she stages regular clinics at each of the apartment towers. The visits are quick, each lasting about fifteen minutes, but are designed to open lines of communication and catch problems early. Lundström says that many seniors will not seek help until a problem is grave enough to warrant a visit to Emergency. Others will have an annual check-up, but will limit themselves strictly to discussing medical matters, ignoring the

---

* It is based on a similar program by the Regional Health Authority in Edmonton.

often more serious emotional component. With a nurse, they are more willing to discuss how they feel overall, and to ask questions about medication, sexuality, and mental health. Unlike what happens with a visit to a physician, many of the seniors will get a follow-up visit at home from the nurse or the therapist.

About 87 per cent of all visits to emergency rooms by seniors are related to falls, so fall prevention is a major focus of the practice. Lundström says she is constantly surprised at how many of her clients use canes or walkers that are inappropriate to their needs. "They buy these things from friends or neighbours, and they are not fitted properly. It's a recipe for disaster," she says. Patients who have mobility problems get a visit from the occupational therapist, and their apartments are modified by volunteer carpenters. There are also a lot of referrals to home care.

Lundström says that one aspect the public-health system has done well is drive home the point that seniors need their blood pressure checked regularly. For many, that is the entry point to the clinic, and the starting point of a preventive-health program. "A lady comes in and says she's fine but just wants her blood pressure checked. But she is so out of breath that I do some checking and realize she has pretty serious cardiac and respiratory difficulties, and I get her to a doctor. Another man comes in for his blood pressure and mentions that he's gained a lot of weight in a short time. It turns out he needs a knee replacement and has stopped taking his long walks, so I get him walking in the pool, and we draw up a plan for his eating, and next thing you know his blood pressure is stabilized. Those are pretty typical of what we see," she says.

When Lundström checks blood pressure at the clinic, she does it twice, once with the patient standing and once with the patient lying down. What the dual reading often reveals is postural hypotension (blood pressure that drops suddenly when a person stands), a common condition that is the leading cause of over-medication in seniors. "If you start with the assumption that most seniors are sick, or have bad hearts, then of course they are going to get a lot of prescriptions. But most of them don't need all the pills they have. The pills cause them more problems than they solve," the nurse says.*

One initiative of the seniors'-health team has been quite effective in reducing medication problems. In conjunction with a nurse, a pharmacist visits a senior, and together they go through the drug cabinet, more often than not revealing expired drugs, overlapping prescriptions, and drug combinations that can be deadly.

Drugs are often a factor in what Lundström calls the "most common and least diagnosed condition among seniors"—depression. She tells of one man who, during a clinic visit, told her he just wanted to lie down in a snowbank and die. He had heart problems and chronic pain, for which he was prescribed morphine, a drug that left him severely depressed. Probing the case with the man, the nurse discovered that the pain was always after meals, that it was caused by gastro-esophageal reflux, not by his heart condition. That meant he didn't need morphine, but treatment for a hiatus hernia. "Once we got past that physical stuff, we tackled depression," Lundström continues. It turns out the man, a dedicated storyteller, could no longer read and write his own stories, and that robbed him of great pleasure. The nurse found him a tape recorder, with which he now records his stories for posterity; his depression has lifted and his health has improved markedly. "Everybody had written him off as dying instead of finding ways of improving his life. That's so typical of the way we treat seniors," Lundström says.

In contrast, she tries to see beyond their bladder problems and backaches, to their wisdom and knowledge. "You have to look beyond the wrinkles to the gold in their veins," Lundström says. For example, she never asks clients their age; she asks, instead, how old they feel. "They often feel younger than they are on paper. That's a sign of good health, and we go from there. As a public-health nurse, you're always trying to find the flicker, the real person

* Research has shown that nurse-practitioners prescribe a fraction of the medication and order a fraction of the tests that family physicians do with comparable patients.

behind all the labels—old person, cardiac patient, disabled—but when you do, it ignites. There's nothing more rewarding."

The key to gerontology, she says, is understanding and treating loss. "As we get older, we all experience losses—driving, friends, your home, maybe your spouse—and they're cumulative. It's no wonder people are depressed, and that it affects their health. They get to feel helpless and hopeless," Lundström says. Giving them hope does not mean magically restoring what was lost, but helping people adapt and adjust. "There is a magic elixir, and it's not a pill, it's giving people control and support. People who are in control are always healthier, regardless of their age."

Lundström and her colleagues try to create that feeling of control on many levels. They instruct in cardiac and stroke prevention; teach bowel and bladder control; help with pain management and sleep hygiene; consult on medication; tackle malnourishment, arthritis, and osteoporosis. But beyond the medical basics, they spend a lot of time on the "giants of geriatrics," caregiver stress and depression. To tackle both, the nurse feels that people need to live in a healthy environment, so she works on building community.

Lundström was born on McKenzie Island, a tiny community near Red Lake, Ontario, that did not even have a hospital. "A lot of my learning comes from living in a small community. People didn't rely on a system, they cared for each other. We lived our lives well because of it," she says. "Now, what I'm doing here is developing these little communities of seniors, these little Red Lakes."

Lundström says that, despite all the attention the seniors'-health team is getting, it is really just a matter of implementing common sense. "This is not revolutionary, this is basic. This is Florence Nightingale unleashing the power of people. We're just doing it with older people, seniors who still have a lot of living left to do."

The I.V. League—Helene Henrichsen

Helene Henrichsen was a highly skilled intravenous nurse working in the high-octane environment at Vancouver General Hospital. Her pager rang constantly as she dashed from department to department, from trauma to organ transplants, installing central lines, Hickman/Broviacs, and other catheters with surgical precision. But when the cuts started coming in 1991, Henrichsen and her colleagues, a roaming team with no department to cling to, were the first to go. "They red-circled us and we were gone," the nurse recalls matter-of-factly.

The trend to jettison IV nurses was widespread. So, Henrichsen answered an ad she saw in the paper for a job at a private clinic. "It was a little scary to be out there without the security of a big hospital umbrella, but I adjusted pretty well," she says. The physician had a small family practice and, on the side, a lucrative intravenous clinic, where most patients came for chelation therapy. The work was pleasant, a far cry from the stressful hospital setting. It also opened her eyes to a whole new world of opportunity. The nurse was earning $35 an hour, while the doctor was bringing in close to seven figures.

Henrichsen realized that, with her skills, she could do this kind of work on her own. But what she lacked was business experience. She approached the Chamber of Commerce and the local Board of Trade. She went back to university to do a certificate in health-care management. Then, in 1993, she took the plunge.

Henrichsen dipped into her savings (largely the pension money she had accumulated at the hospital) and purchased a handful of reclining chairs that she set up in the living room of her home. The patients started trickling in to the new business, which was given a catchy name: The I.V. League Inc. "Pretty soon we outgrew the place. It was a bit much for the family to have patients in the living room all the time," the nurse says.

Henrichsen looked at space in medical buildings, but the rent was exorbitant. She opted instead to buy a big old house, where one floor could be dedicated solely to business. It is wheelchair-accessible, and has plenty of parking and a bus stop right out front. And now there are nine recliners. But the clinic has a homey feel, with classical music playing, and fruit and juices laid out for the patients. "It's important to me that they feel safe and comfortable here. I don't just poke my patients, I care for them," she says.

The first client arrives around 7:00 A.M., and the last one usually leaves by 3:00 P.M. Most of the IV drips infuse over several hours, so patients read, eat, and often nap in their recliners. Henrichsen inserts all the IVs herself, as well as charting. She opens the clinic four days a week, and does one night and another day of home visits.

Henrichsen's bread and butter is chelation therapy. It is a process in which patients receive, by intravenous drip, artificial amino acid and vitamins that remove substances from tissue. The bulk of her patients are in their sixties and seventies, and have heart and circulatory problems. Many are not healthy enough for surgery, or they want to take action while on waiting lists. They hope the treatment will remove plaque from their arteries. The process is controversial—some researchers claim it does nothing for arteriosclerosis—but it is a popular alternative treatment in B.C.

Henrichsen, who has studied chelation therapy extensively, defends it as a legitimate treatment, but does not tout it as a miracle cure. "This is a slow process, it takes time. I tell lots of people who come here to go back to their doctor and get a bypass or angioplasty. But many of them can't or won't," she says. She takes great pride in the fact that most of her clients have been elsewhere, but tend to stick with her. "These patients are quite sick and they are very vulnerable. There are a lot of charlatans out there. They trust a nurse. They know they're going to get straight answers and good care," she says.

An initial course of chelation treatment consists of about thirty visits at $85, then maintenance of six visits annually. Henrichsen likes the fact that, with repeat visits, she gets to know clients quite well, a stark contrast to her hospital work. What is a little more difficult is that chelation is not covered by medicare, nor by most private insurance plans, so patients must pay for it themselves. Chelation therapy is, however, tax-deductible as a medical expense. "Most of my clients are well-to-do, they can afford it and it's not a hardship at all. But, yes, it bothers me that the service is not available to everyone," she says.

Aside from chelation therapy, Henrichsen does some antibiotic treatments, many on contract for the Workers' Compensation Board. Some chemotherapy patients will also come to her when they are travelling, because they want to avoid a hospital setting, or to get additional multivitamin treatments. She is also the nurse of choice for very wealthy business people and movie stars who want to be visited on the quiet in their hotel suites, for treatments ranging from vitamins to chemotherapy. "These are clients who can afford anything, and they choose to have a nurse do their IVs. I think that should tell us something about nursing," Henrichsen says.

Although business is booming in the IV field, she has chosen not to extend clinic hours and hire other nurses, preferring a hands-on practice. In total, the IV nurse sees thirty to forty clients a week. "I'm not big, I don't see hundreds of people a week like some clinics. I try to offer quality and a personal touch, and I'm very protective of my clients," she says. Rather than expand, Henrichsen's idea is to franchise "The I.V. League," and to create a network of small, homey intravenous clinics around the country. But she is not ready yet.

"I think I'm a typical nurse in the sense that I'm not a risk-taker. We like to do our jobs well, not to seek out glory," Henrichsen says. Still, she did gamble by going into business, and it has paid off. Her home business grosses more than $100,000 a year. "I'm certainly not rich. I make a little more than I would at the hospital, but I feel a lot better about it. I feel respected. I didn't feel that way as a hospital nurse."

The hardest part of being an entrepreneur, Henrichsen says, is the lack of supports, having to do it all alone. Sticking a needle into the vein of a jaundiced, emaciated patient with circulatory problems is never easy, but knowing there is no one to back you up adds pressure. But, on the other hand, she says, in the clinic she can take all the time she needs, and use heat packs and other tricks, because there aren't impatient surgeons hovering.

Henrichsen's only employee is a secretary. That means the nurse has to do all the chores herself, including buying supplies, doing the bookkeeping, and site maintenance, which involves scrubbing the floors every night. "At the hospital, you just leave at the end of the day. What's exhausting here is all the little stuff you have to do when the clients aren't around," she says.

But the biggest adjustment for her was working alone, in a laid-back atmosphere. "I've always done acute nursing, crisis management. I miss that a bit, but what I miss most of all is my comrades. Nursing is a very social profession and, in contrast, being in business can be very lonely." The IV team at Vancouver General, for example, was very close and, almost a decade after it was disbanded, the women stay in touch. Today, they have their parties at The I.V. League.

Henrichsen says she gets a lot of calls from fed-up nurses who are intrigued by entrepreneurship and are looking for advice. "I tell them that it's not as easy as they think to run a successful business, but it's worth it."

At age 50, when many nurses are thinking about retirement, she is rejuvenated by new challenges. "If I was still at the hospital, I think my career would be almost over. But I'm certainly not going to retire now. I love what I'm doing and plan to continue for a long time," Henrichsen says.

In fact, if the IV nurse has one regret, it is not having made the leap to private enterprise sooner. "Look at me, I'm just a nurse— a fat little old nurse—and I've done this. I'm successful and I'm happy. I'm not saying it was easy, but nurses have this ability to learn, to adapt, and they have to realize just how valuable that is in the world outside the hospital."

The Special Moments—Roxanne MacLeod

Married for fifty-five years, the couple had always made a point of doing something memorable on New Year's Eve. But this year he was dying, in the terminal phase of cancer, and she was grieving. But when palliative-home-care nurse Roxanne MacLeod arrived at their Charlottetown home for her shift, a quick decision was made to continue the tradition. The two women rounded up candles, dimmed the lights, and put the couple's favourite music on the stereo. The wife climbed into bed and snuggled her husband tight, swaying gently to the melodies and falling asleep in his arms one last time.

"When you work in palliative care, it's important to create those private, special moments. When people are at home, there's an intimacy that you can't get in a hospital," MacLeod says. There is a growing realization that hospitals are for sick people, not necessarily for those who are dying.

When she started working at the private home-care agency We Care Home Health Services Inc., in 1996, only a fraction of clientele wanted to die at home. Today, almost 40 per cent of the company's business is palliative. Across Canada, the demand for palliative home care is growing at a similar pace, for a number of reasons.* Due to cutbacks, it is more difficult, and less pleasant, to remain in hospital, even for a patient who is seriously ill. Word-of-mouth is an important factor, as the vast majority of families have a positive home-care experience. Further, perceptions about the role of the health-care system are shifting to the view that proper care consists of much more than treating specific diseases; rather, it begins with prevention and ends with ensuring a comfortable death. Palliative care is leading the way, as one of the few mainstream programs that takes a holistic approach.

The major drawback is financial. In more provinces than not,

* About 20 per cent of Canadians die at home, but polls show that more than 80 per cent would opt to do so if proper supports were in place.

families must pay for palliative home care themselves: not only for nursing, but for medical supplies, for equipment rental, and even for beds that would all be provided free of charge if the patient chose to die in hospital.

"For me as a nurse, it's very frustrating to know that we turn people down because they don't have the means. It's a big flaw in the system to say that we will pay all the costs in the hospital, no matter how high, but we won't help people at all who want to spend their last days in the privacy and comfort of their homes," MacLeod says.*

There is significant cost to nurses too. To keep their fees down, home-care agencies pay about $7 an hour less than nurses earn in a hospital setting. (Generally, there is not an appreciable difference between the wages paid by non-profit and for-profit agencies in the community. But some provinces, such as British Columbia and Saskatchewan, use the same pay scale for institutional and community nurses.)

MacLeod says that the ready acceptance of lower wages for community-based workers is insulting, but it is a reflection of society's undervaluing of care. The system itself also perpetuates discrimination. When she studied for her diploma at the P.E.I. College of Nursing, the focus was entirely on acute care, and nursing jobs in Emergency and Intensive Care were held up as the pinnacle of the profession. It was not until MacLeod began studying for her baccalaureate at Dalhousie University that she discovered the importance of community nursing. Yet, despite the markedly lower pay, MacLeod may have had the last laugh; since graduating in 1993, she has always had full-time work in home care, but virtually all her classmates, who pursued the institutional acute-care route, have been juggling casual jobs. MacLeod says she has also been lucky to land a job at We Care, a company that is Canada's greatest nursing entrepreneurship success story. (Founded

---

* A 1999 study found that home care saves, on average, $8,000 a year per case, regardless of the level of care required.

by nurse Bev McMaster in Brandon, Manitoba, in 1984, We Care is now the largest independent home-care company in the country. Each of its eighty franchises is nurse-owned, and there are almost 5,000 employees in total.)

Aside from pay, the most difficult aspect of palliative-home-care nursing is that it is lonely and isolating. MacLeod carries out all the tasks the client needs alone, including medical care, personal care, making the bed, and even meal preparation—"and we didn't have cooking classes in nursing school," she quips. "But seriously, the thing I love about palliative care in the home setting is that you care for every aspect of the family's needs: physical, emotional, and spiritual. You build relationships in the way you can never do in a hospital."

Clients who need home care for a few weeks after surgery, or those who need long-term chronic care, tend to purchase set blocks of services, from thirty minutes to twelve hours a day of nursing care, supplemented by homemaking services. In those instances, a nurse can see up to ten clients daily. (Nurses also supervise the homemaking staff and personal-care attendants.)

In palliative care, nurses will often work exclusively with one patient, with daily shifts of eight or twelve hours. This is designed to ensure continuity and to allow families to feel more comfortable with care providers. The "active dying" phase—when treatments are no longer effective—can range from several months down to a couple of weeks. "Seeing the same faces all the time is essential for the families because it builds trust. It's really such an invasion, going into a person's home for twenty-four hours a day, that you want them to be as comfortable as possible with you," MacLeod says.

There is no set routine for nursing care, but there are priorities. Regular skin care and moving of patients is essential to avoid bed sores, infections that can prove fatal for those with compromised immune systems. MacLeod places a lot of emphasis on encouraging patients to socialize, and will change her plans to make it easier for friends and family to visit. "One of the good things about dying at home is that a lot more people will visit than at the hospital. It's not as depressing." Pain management is also a focus, and MacLeod uses a full gamut of techniques, including drugs, massage, music, and therapeutic touch.

When a new patient is taken on for palliative care, one of the first things the nurse will do with family members is rearrange the house to make it more comfortable for the patient. A hospital bed needs to be rented or purchased, along with medical aids and equipment such as a walker, a catheter, an intravenous stand, a hydraulic lift, an oxygen-saturation monitor, and, in some instances, a ventilator. Essentially, the nurse creates a mini ICU. MacLeod recommends keeping all the technology in one room so families can maintain control of their homes. Most palliative patients opt to move into the living room. It tends to be the brightest room; it is usually on the ground floor (no stairs); and it is usually the hub of activity in the home, keeping the dying person at the centre of family life, not hidden away in a backroom. The smell of your coffee, the sight of the dog sleeping nearby, and the overheard telephone conversations are little snippets of life that create stability and normalcy, even for a dying person.

MacLeod also invests a lot of time in teaching families how to care because it helps them feel more in control. "It can all be overwhelming to the family, especially if they're just sitting back watching the nurse and feeling helpless. Helping out with things, even adjusting the bed or assisting with a bath can make people feel really good. They become a caregiver, not just a spectator."

But living, breathing, and eating with a dying person twenty-four hours a day for weeks or months on end can take its toll. Sometimes family members just can't take it anymore, especially when the patient has difficulty controlling the pain (as is the case with some cancers and neurological diseases). MacLeod teaches them from day one that there is no shame in going to hospital, that comfort always comes first.

Where problems sometimes arise for the nurse is when a patient has made it perfectly clear that he or she wants to die at home and does not want extraordinary measures taken, and a family member panics. "Most palliative deaths are quite predictable. You know exactly what's going to happen. But, if at the end, someone says: 'Take him to the hospital now. Save him,' and you know that contradicts the patient's wishes, it can be a huge ethical and moral dilemma. Luckily, that hardly ever happens. We make sure the family is prepared," MacLeod says.

The nurse has the power to pronounce death, but confirms that with a physician by phone. (The coroner does not have to be contacted for predictable palliative deaths.) MacLeod makes arrangements with the funeral home to transport the corpse. She also prepares the body, removing the catheter and IV, putting on glasses and dentures, and changing the sheets and clothes. If the family wishes, she will pray with them. "And I always make tea or coffee because that provides a distraction," MacLeod notes.

Many families will keep the body at home for several hours, so people can say their goodbyes. The nurse stays to offer comfort and counselling. In most instances, she also makes phone calls to inform other family members of the death. "Again, the atmosphere is different at home. You have the freedom to grieve on your own terms. If you want to pray over the body for hours, or if you want to cry out loud, you can do it, and there won't be fifteen people coming in and out of the room. At home, you have the death you want, on your terms."

No One Else Left to Care — Madeleine Shorthill

As long-term-care facilities go, Mount Tolmie Hospital in Victoria is as nice as they come. Completely renovated a decade ago, it still looks brand new, with wide, sparkling corridors leading, spokelike, to a sunny central courtyard. What gives it an institutional feel is the fact that all the rooms are quads and doubles. "This four-to-a-room concept harkens back to a different time. Personally, I think everyone deserves a private room. That change is coming because consumers are demanding it, but it comes down to money," says Madeleine Shorthill, the nursing team leader at the facility.

Much change has already come to the long-term-care sector. To save money, many seniors with health problems remain in the community, with varying levels of home care. That means patients residing in facilities arrive much later in life, with far more acute health-care problems. At Mount Tolmie, for example, more than half of patients have some form of dementia, most in advanced stages, and as many again have serious physical disabilities, with the combination being increasingly frequent. Many patients have Alzheimer's, Parkinson's, or grave health problems related to strokes and heart disease. "The reality is that someone coming here is coming for the rest of their life," Shorthill says. The average stay is now less than eighteen months, down from about five years, since cutbacks.

"Patients don't come here to die. They come here to live the rest of their lives as comfortably as possible. There's an important distinction," Shorthill says. The difference is the level and quality of care. "Our philosophy is that residents have a right to make choices, to make their own decisions, and we are there to help. We believe people have the right to end their lives in a dignified manner."

Providing all the care and nurturing that the acutely ill require, however, is sometimes difficult. Like everywhere else in the hospital sector, there have been big cuts, many of them affecting nurses. At Mount Tolmie, a seventy-three-bed facility that is always full, there is only one registered nurse on the overnight shift. This is not unusual at all anymore; nursing homes often have a single nurse for 100 patients; and some patients go through extended periods of the day without a professional nurse. Asked if the ratio of nurses to patients is adequate, Shorthill chooses her words carefully. "I don't hesitate to say care is good," she says, pausing. "Nor do I hesitate to say it could be improved. There are times when professional nursing input is thin on the ground, and that is worrisome. If there was a budget for more professional nurses, we could use them, and I believe that is true of all long-term-care facilities."

The reality is that most tasks are now carried out by nursing assistants, and the nurse's role is to coordinate care. Assistants do basic hygiene such as bathing, help residents with dressing and toileting, change the beds, and help patients eat. Residents of long-term-care facilities, no matter their physical and mental disabilities, are now rarely bed-bound. Assistants, using various mechanical aids, are also responsible for getting them out and about. "At an extended-care facility, you don't need a nurse doing that. What you need is a professional supervising care to ensure that it is done correctly," Shorthill says.

She notes, too, that at Mount Tolmie only professional nurses dispense medications, give injections, do dressings, and monitor high-technology equipment such as respirators. So, during the day, there will be a half-dozen nurses, a stark contrast to the staffing at some private facilities.

Shorthill's role is planning for admissions, staffing, supervising the nursing and non-nursing staff, and a lot of troubleshooting. Admissions are quite different here from what occurs in most hospital settings, for a number of reasons. Mount Tolmie, because it has a good reputation, has a long waiting list, so patients can wait anywhere from months to a year for a bed. Caregivers are obviously quite stressed during this waiting period, and when admission time comes a different emotion takes over. There is a certain finality and a significant cost* associated with admission to a long-term-care facility these days, and that often leads to a lot of guilt for family members. "When we admit a patient, we say that we're admitting the family too, and they sometimes need as much care to deal with their conflicting emotions," Shorthill says.

Change, particularly for people with forms of dementia, can be disruptive and upsetting. For those coming from a home setting, as is increasingly frequent, the adaptation to an institutional setting, notably four-to-a-room accommodation, can also be very

---

* Even a public hospital like Mount Tolmie charges about $1,400 a month (about one-third of actual costs), reasoning that the charge is for room and board, not for medical services.

difficult. That often translates into inappropriate behaviours or anger towards staff. Shorthill also has to keep families up to date on the condition of their loved ones. To this end, there are routine resident reviews, conducted by a multidisciplinary team, and including family, a process that takes a lot of organizational work.

Patients, too, are requiring more managerial care. The nurse says that the stereotype of meek, compliant elderly is not at all accurate, and that many patients do not hesitate to question policy and demand changes. "Be careful not to be fooled by their outward appearance," Shorthill warns. "That 'poor little old man' in the wheelchair over there headed a university. He's a brilliant scholar, and he can make his opinions known quite eloquently." Shorthill welcomes the change, the consumer awareness, but again warns that it will have policy implications down the road. For example, she sees patients demanding a greater presence of professional nurses.

Yet, in this era of shortages, the most time-consuming and demanding part of Shorthill's job is filling the jobs that now exist. Attracting staff to gerontology has long been a challenge, and doubly so for shift work in long-term-care facilities. "Nursing homes have an image problem. A lot of nurses out there think extended care is the bottom of the heap," she says. "The saving grace is that, once they're here, those who give it a chance dramatically and quickly change their minds. This is one of the most neglected and ignored groups in society, and it's rewarding to work with them because they need you so badly."

Still, Shorthill says care is beginning to suffer because she finds it virtually impossible to find replacements on holidays and educational days. That, in turn, makes the full-time jobs less appealing. "If you have a family and are told that holidays in July or August are out of the question, and that each time someone is sick you have to pick up an extra shift, you're not going to be happy, and you're not going to stick around," she says dejectedly. Shorthill does not believe lives are at risk, but rather that nurses no longer have time for the "niceties" that distinguish their caregiving from the services of all other health professionals.

"People should not care about shortages because they make my job more difficult. They should care profoundly because the bottom line is that residents and their families are the big losers when there is a nursing shortage. When there are no nurses, there is no one else left to care."

Lest We Remember—Merial Forde

People do not die of Alzheimer's disease. Rather, they die a thousand little deaths as the debilitating neurological disease robs them of their ability to carry out the simple tasks of daily life, and plunges them into a jumbled and often frightening morass of memories. For veterans, those men who fought in the bloody conflicts of the First and Second World Wars and Korea, these remembrances can be a cruel form of torture, a never-ending reliving of long-ago horrors.

"These guys are different from other Alzheimer's patients, from other patients with dementia. The war is always uppermost in their minds, and any little gesture you make can be a trigger," says Merial Forde, a nurse in the special-care ward for veterans at Parkwood Hospital* in London, Ontario. "Because of this, you need strategies, even for bath time. Normally, water is comforting, but for veterans it has a lot of meaning—perhaps a river long ago, infested with snakes or crocodiles, or a rain storm beating down on fallen comrades during a bloody battle."

As Forde explains her work, how the seemingly simple tasks are impregnated with meaning, she betrays a profound empathy for her patients, and an intimate knowledge that comes from caring for the same people for many years. For one man,† showering is out of the question, it is too frightening; another needs his hair washed so that no water gets in his ears; yet another loves to linger

---

* A freestanding long-term-care centre, it is now administered by St. Joseph's Health Centre, but much of the funding comes from Veterans Affairs.
† There are women veterans, but they are a minority, and Forde does not have any in her care.

in the water, to let himself float away. "My guys," she calls them. And they, in turn, call her "my nurse."

In the nursing model employed by Parkwood, one registered nurse cares for five veterans. Each patient has a private room. On each door is the patient's name, and a photo, usually of a strapping young man in dress uniform. There are many more photos on each wall. There is a garden, and a lounge, and a long hallway featuring a "race track." (Because many Alzheimer's patients like to pace obsessively, many facilities now instal tracks in the hallway, with a rail down the middle. The rail gives them support, and keeps them apart to prevent jostling.)

Forde's patients range in age from 78 to 89. They were not only soldiers, but company executives, professional athletes, and labourers.* In addition to dementia, some have mental illnesses such as schizophrenia or physical conditions such as diabetes and chronic lung disease. The only prerequisite for veterans is that they be ambulatory. The nurse knows all the names of their children, details of their jobs, even the units they served in during the war. Knowing their past is essential to understanding their present.

At Parkwood, nurses perform many tasks that elsewhere are carried out by nursing assistants and orderlies. Familiar faces are important to patients, and specialized knowledge is needed to understand the mood and condition of the patients.

Forde's day begins at 7:30 A.M. with a report. Morning care is among the most difficult. Although it consists of helping the men get washed and dressed, "it can be a real challenge if they're not in that time and space," she says. It is physically demanding, sometimes likened to caring for a 100-kilogram baby. The nurse helps her patients get to breakfast, and feeds some. There are morning meds and continence pads to be changed. Patients have morning appointments with dentists, doctors, and classes such as art therapy. Though there are porters, nurses will often do transport because it is less upsetting for patients. There is a snack, lunch, and

* To ensure their privacy, only the barest of details are being provided.

another change, then many patients have a nap. Nurses then get started on documentation, which is extensive. "You have flow sheets for infection, evacuation, how they eat, how they walk, daily hygiene, everything. Because patients can't remember anything, we write it all down. There's lots of paperwork," Forde says.

At 3:00 P.M., another shift comes in, so there is some overlap. Afternoon is also an active time. Many Alzheimer's patients demonstrate "sundown behaviour," a burst of activity, and for many that occurs around 3:00 P.M. and/or 3:00 A.M. (The race track is always crowded between 3:00 A.M. and 4:00 A.M.) This is often a time of conflict. "Being men and being veterans, things happen. There are altercations, verbal and physical, all the time," Forde says. Nurses are usually in the middle of them, and take more than their share of punches, kicks, and blows from canes. "You just get in there; you don't think of the danger, you just try to stop them from hurting each other," says Forde, a tall, strong woman who has the advantage of towering over some of the men.

Before dinner, there is a snack, another round of meds, and another change. Then, before her shift ends at 7:30 P.M., Forde gets her guys ready for bed. "When I go through my day hour by hour, it doesn't sound like very much. It's hard for a nurse to tell you what happens. It's a steady barrage, a whole bunch of little things, and they all add up to care. You're, first and foremost, a caregiver, but you're also a social worker, referee, porter, a shoulder to cry on. You can't do these things justice writing them down," she says.

After thirty years as a nurse, the past twenty at Parkwood, Forde seems to carry out her duties effortlessly. But it infuriates her when people confuse that ease with easiness. Parkwood, she says, knows the value of professional nurses, and she fumes when she hears of institutions replacing nurses with nursing assistants and technicians. "Take something that looks simple, like feeding. Some of my guys 'forget' to swallow, or they 'forget' that they're hungry. You need to understand body knowledge, you need experience, to get them through a meal. Having untrained people here would be dangerous," she says.

In fact, a key part of a nurse's work in a long-term-care facility is constant assessment: breathing patterns, skin changes, abrasions, moods. A veteran like Forde, while she is chatting with the men, checks their nails for clues on oxygenation of their blood, gets an idea of the condition of their circulatory system from new bruises, spots rashes that can be indicative of scabies or infections, and notices mood swings and changes in sleeping patterns that might show a new medication is not appropriate.

"When outsiders see nurses chatting, they think it's an easy job. They don't understand that we're scanning, we're assessing, we're learning. We have to get a patient who can't tell us anything to tell us everything that's going on in his body and his mind," the nurse says.

She does not buy into the common belief that gerontology is at the bottom of the nursing scale. On the contrary, Forde says, nurses in the specialty have a lot more say and a lot more control than those in "sexier" areas such as pediatrics. "We have input into everything on the ward, right down to the type of furniture."

Having five patients to care for full-time is something that other nurses envy, and rightfully so, says Forde, because she gets to build close and lasting relationships with the men and their families. Some, after all, have been in her care for almost a decade.

The hardest part of the work is not the patients themselves, but helping their families grieve. Forde tells of one patient, very dignified and impeccably dressed, who would spend hours on his hands and knees, scrubbing the floor with a toothbrush (he was reliving a job he had as a cleaner before he became very successful in business). The man's wife was mortified and ashamed until, one day, their son got down on his hands and knees too, determined to spend time with his dad, to enter his world again, by whatever means possible. The father smiled, and the mother beamed with pride, Forde says, her eyes welling up with tears at the memory.

"People think it's a terrible thing to be locked in with these guys, but it's not. Even though they're demented, there are windows when you see the real person, the social graces, the humour, the intelligence, the wonderful lives they've had. I always tell the families, yes, it's a horrible disease, but grasp the good things, savour those moments."

It is not only advice, but a philosophy Forde lives by. In her early fifties, she is preparing to retire, determined to savour the time she has left. Physically, she's in good shape, but, like so many nurses today, she is mentally exhausted. Forde, who started her career in pediatrics and will end it in geriatrics, plans to close the circle in retirement. She intends to use her free time volunteering in schools, in particular, to assist children with special needs integrate, and to help people in the community understand increasingly common conditions such as dementia.

"I will never stop being a nurse. My skills will not be lost, they will just be used differently."

A Good Death — Carolyn Adams

The first thing Carolyn Adams does when she walks in to a patient's room is sit down at the bedside. This is unusual, because many hospital nurses don't get off their feet once in a twelve-hour shift. But in palliative care it sends an important message. "When I sit down, I'm telling the patients that I'm not in a hurry to rush out. I'm there for them. I'm there to listen, to help them get through that day."

Palliative-care nurses such as those at Royal Victoria Hospital in Montreal are not miracle workers. They cannot keep death at bay, but they can help gravely ill patients have, in the parlance of hospice care, a "good death." That means, above all, that the patient has some control.

Palliative care used to consist of letting people die and providing some pain relief. Today, nurses and physicians intervene much more actively. For example, a woman with bone cancer might get a hip replacement for pain relief, even though she can no longer be treated with chemotherapy or radiation therapy. "We do whatever is appropriate for comfort—surgery, medication, massage, whatever.

It's a bit of a cliché, but palliative care is not about dying, it's about living today. Yes, death will come eventually, but we help patients enjoy the rest of their lives as fully and comfortably as possible. Our work isn't just technical, it's emotional and spiritual too," Adams says.

When she comes in for her shift at 7:30 A.M. each day, there is a quick report, reading of charts, and preparation of medications. Shifts are eight hours, and each nurse is assigned four patients. But as soon as her patients awake, she is taking a seat at bedside. The purpose of those chats is to set priorities for the day. The nurse is not only a caregiver, but a coordinator of everything from family visits to medication.

A patient may want a bath and massage for pain relief. Adams will do that herself, saying it is one of her most cherished tasks. "Touch is so important. When they feel my hands, they know I care." Bathing and massage are also so intimate that they often get patients talking. "A lot comes out. You learn a lot during bath time, and the more you learn, the better care you can provide," she says.

Adams often plays classical music during bath time. In fact, quiet music wafts continually across the ward. There is a CD and cassette library, and a piano. Songs evoke memories, and music is often associated with happy times. The music therapist does regular rounds, as does the pet therapist. There are also a lot of volunteers (one is assigned to each nurse on each shift), who help with chores like feeding, and act as a listening post.

They try to bring a sense of normalcy to the lives of those who are dying. The lounge, a solarium that looks out onto beautiful Mount Royal, is the site for group events: coffee time on Tuesday and Thursday, wine and cheese on Wednesday, live music on Sunday, and other special occasions such as weddings, baptisms, birthdays, and Christmas parties. Normalcy also means involving families, and much of the work of the palliative-care nurse centres on the family. Preparing loved ones for death is often more work than preparing the patient. This is particularly true in light of the changing family structure: the dynamics of ex-husbands, stepchildren, multiple grandparents, and estranged lovers can be a challenge to the most diplomatic nurse.

"Lots of families say: 'Don't tell my mom, she doesn't know she's dying.' Our experience is that Mom knows very well what's going on, and it's the adult children who are having trouble. Sometimes you have angry families who lash out at the nurses. They're frightened, struggling with their own emotions, and looking for someone to blame. Other times, there are family feuds that play themselves out," Adams explains.

Caring for the terminally ill is emotional work. Patients are urged, before it is too late, to say what they have to say, to make their peace. That results in a lot of heart-wrenching talks. Nurses are there to facilitate, to ensure patients are able to tell their family members and friends what they want to, be it in person or in a letter, or by making a farewell video (an increasingly popular option in the video age).

Adams relates the story of a woman who asked to see her daughters because she had something important to say. "When they got there, she said: 'I don't want you there when I die.' They couldn't believe it. But she started telling them how she was never there for them as a mother, how she had failed, and she didn't deserve their support now. It was all really heartbreaking." But, despite her advanced condition, the woman had a dramatic turnaround and lived another year. "Because of that talk, she ended up having a relationship with her daughters that she never had."

Patients are also urged to bring in mementos, to make their rooms as homey as possible. One woman attached a mural, a picture of a starry sky, with one star shining particularly brightly, to the ceiling above her bed. "One day, just before she died, her grandson was cuddling on the bed with her and she said: 'You see that star? That's me. After I'm gone, you will be able to see me every night.'" It is those once-in-a-lifetime moments, Adams says, that make palliative-care nursing such a privilege.

A long-time gerontology and oncology nurse, she became interested in palliative care after her own grandfather became one of her patients, and died on her ward. "I was trying to deal with him as a granddaughter and as a chemotherapy nurse. I was wearing many hats and saw the death from every side. But it wasn't a good death. Grandpa was scared, I was overwhelmed, and we didn't get the support we needed. It was devastating," she says.

As part of her grieving, Adams learned about palliative care, and she came to understand its importance. Before that point, she, like a lot of nurses, knew only that nurses were supposed to get people well and back into the community. But she realized that was not always going to happen, and nurses have an important role in preparing patients for death too.

Fortunately, there have been major advances in understanding pain and how to control it. There are many drugs aside from morphine. Epidurals are now fairly common in palliative care; so are syringe drivers, which allow medication to be infused subcutaneously over a twenty-four-hour period. Patients are turned regularly, and there are all kinds of new equipment, such as state-of the-art mattresses, which prevent bed sores, a common source of discomfort. Patients, even those who are actively dying, are also hydrated but, again, subcutaneously instead of intravenously, to reduce pain. In fact, a regular part of the nurses' routine is distributing pain medication on schedule, and monitoring patients who need treatment for breakthrough pain. The only physical pain that remains difficult to control is neuropathic (in the peripheral nerves).

Palliative-care nurses routinely deal with death. In the sixteen-bed ward at the Royal Vic, there will be up to three deaths daily. That can be draining. Adams is deeply religious—a born-again Christian—and says that helps her cope. "I've also learned to take better care of my own physical and emotional health. That keeps it from being overwhelming. You also pace yourself. I have two boys and I make sure they don't get emotional leftovers," she says.

The moment of death is one of the most significant parts of Adams's work. She recognizes that it's important that people not die alone, that they have their loved ones with them. It's also important for nurses to be there to complete the powerful journey with their patients. Adams says that she often knows that a death has been a good one based on the reaction of the family. "If we've handled things well, they get through a lot of the grieving beforehand. When death comes, it's not like a bomb has dropped, it's more like a candle that has been blown out. When a family leaves here at peace, I know I've done a good job, I know I've made a difference."

Part Eight
NURSING
AND BEYOND

The World's a Stage

For decades, women chose nursing because it was the best of limited job options, work that they could do until they were married and had children, and that they could take up again after the children grew up. Today, nursing is not merely a job, it is a career choice. Those who choose nursing want, like other professionals, the ability to advance, to find new challenges, as their careers progress. Until recently, those opportunities have been quite restricted: the role of the nurse was limited, and those who aspired to more would quickly hit a glass ceiling at the head-nurse level. Today, however, that is all changing. Practice guidelines are expanding rapidly; there are dozens of nursing specialties to pursue in institutional and community settings; and opportunities are burgeoning for entrepreneurs in research and in health-care management.

As nursing gains respect as an independent profession and expands into uncharted territory, many nurses are emerging as leaders, charting a course in administration, influencing health policy both domestically and internationally, and helping shape the political agenda. While many of these women are removed from hands-on patient care, they are unanimous in saying that a nursing background has a profound influence on how they do their jobs. In fact, it was only by stepping away that many of them came to truly appreciate the joys of nursing, and the opportunities it opened to them.

Many of the nurses featured in *Critical Care*, and particularly those in Part Eight, who are recognized as among the leaders in the profession in Canada, are following in the footsteps of Florence Nightingale. During the Crimean War, Nightingale instituted basic rules of hygiene and professionalism that forever changed nursing, hospitals and, ultimately, medicine. While the image of the benevolent lady with the lamp is a lasting one, it is but a fraction of what she stood for and achieved during a fifty-year career as a scholar, researcher, educator, policy analyst, and savvy lobbyist.

One of Nightingale's rightful heirs is Red Cross worker Élisabeth Carrier (though, for the record, it should be noted that Nightingale was a fierce critic of the Red Cross, in large part because their delegates were laymen, not medical professionals such as nurses and doctors). Carrier has been an eyewitness to some of the worst acts of savagery in history, including the killing fields of Cambodia and the Rwandan genocide. On her many missions, she not only provided medical assistance, but promoted human rights and offered basic aid, including such necessities as food and water. Recently, Carrier has moved to the position of International Red Cross delegate, responsible for verifying adherence to the principles of the Geneva Convention, a role in which her ability to do critical analysis is invaluable.

Rose Reynolds Nakatsuru discovered early in her career that a nursing degree can now take you in many directions. Working with a number of community groups during her studies steered her towards the charitable world, where she works for a foundation and oversees the disbursement of more than $1 million annually in health-care research grants. Like Nightingale, Reynolds sets her focus on the environmental, not medical, aspects of health, on pursuing commonsense solutions to contemporary health problems.

Margaret Hilson of the Canadian Public Health Association has also used her nursing skills in ways few would dream of. A living legend in the international-development world, she has taken a fundamental premise of nursing—that everyone deserves basic care—and applied it on a global scale. Like Nightingale, Hilson has greatly influenced, and been greatly influenced by, the community health-care model in India. And Nightingale's once-radical view that you cannot simply transplant a Western health-care model into a developing country has been a guiding principle of her career. She readily admits that, after so many years away from the medical side, she is not qualified to administer direct care to patients. But Hilson stubbornly insists that she is a nurse because that is the philosophical underpinning of all her policy-development initiatives, work that will influence the way health care is delivered to millions of people.

After the Crimean War, Nightingale turned her mind to hospital design, producing the book *Notes on Hospitals*. With that work, she revolutionized the institution by proposing that hospitals be not only airy and clean (they were, until that time, largely dank and rat-infested), but organized into units, or pavilions, that minimized the spread of disease and placed emphasis on specialization.

Mary Ferguson-Paré, the vice-president of massive Vancouver Hospital, is following Nightingale's model as one of North America's foremost experts on organizational management in the health-care field. She has rocketed up the management ladder with a combination of higher education, superior people skills, and the no-nonsense approach she learned as a psychiatric nurse. Today, the fundamental role for hospitals is not controlling infection but creating patient-centred care, and Ferguson-Paré feels the way to achieve that is to provide more nursing care, and to give nurses greater leeway to practise independently. As a senior administrator, she has demonstrated the influence that nurses can have when they use their skills to forge policy. Creating a better workplace is essential not only to patients, but also to keeping nurses on the job.

The frustrations of working in the Canadian health system have led many to look for better opportunities. For those with specialized skills such as intensive-care or pediatric cardiology, the lure can be hard to resist. Sadly, it is often the best and brightest who go first, particularly to the United States.* Some nurses have taken advantage of the brain drain. Linda Beechinor makes a good living as a full-time nurse recruiter, wooing hundreds of her fellow Canadians to the island paradise of Hawaii. Nurses there have better pay, as well as better working conditions. And, as recruiters back in Canada know, money is rarely the motivating factor for nurses making a move. They are looking for full-time work (which is difficult to find in these days of casualization) and the ability to build a career, by upgrading education, and for jobs that promise some regularity. And the longer nurses stay away, the less likely they are to return to Canada.

When Florence Nightingale returned to England after the Crimean War, she did so under an assumed name, determined to avoid the spotlight and pursue scholarly research. As a folk hero, the nurse could have pursued any opportunity she wanted, but chose to work anonymously in government, as the principal investigator for a royal commission investigating health in the British Army.

Judith Shamian, a nursing administrator and researcher whose work is known internationally, has chosen a similarly unconventional route. At the height of her career, as she was being solicited to head a major teaching hospital, she opted instead to take up a newly created post at Health Canada: executive director of nursing policy. As a long-time head of nursing at Mount Sinai Hospital in Toronto, she spent years grappling with the problem of staff shortages. Now, as the country's new "head nurse," she will turn her attention full time to seeking answers, and averting the potentially grave crisis that could occur should projections prove correct.

Shamian is convinced that a made-in-Canada solution is necessary. The nurses who seek fame and fortune abroad make the headlines, but, even if they were to all come home, they would barely make a dent in the shortfalls. On the other hand, there are probably as many nurses in Canada who are no longer working in

* A recent study found that about one-third of new graduates leave Canadian nursing within three years of graduation. About 10 percent migrate to the U.S., and more than 20 percent leave for other jobs in the health-care sector.

the field as there are who are still working in it. This is a great untapped resource. One of Shamian's first goals is to figure out where these women have gone, and why. She has anecdotal evidence that working conditions have to improve and that more opportunities for advancement need to exist.

In the wave of cutbacks, one of the first positions to go was that of head nurse. This middle-management position was not only a managerial training ground, but also an anchor for staff nurses, who now have to deal with human-resource managers rather than with peers who share their professional background. Many nurses have left the traditional hospital setting to become entrepreneurs. Many more have left to pursue careers in other fields.

A number of the nurses featured in *Critical Care* have had handsome offers from the private sector, but chose to remain with their first love, publicly funded health care, despite the paltry salaries and lack of perks. A skilled nurse-researcher can double her or his salary overnight by jumping to a pharmaceutical company; a manager can do the same by accepting an offer from one of the growing number of private health-care agencies. It is surprising to discover just how many senior business leaders, policy analysts, and politicians (including a handful of provincial Health ministers) have nursing backgrounds.

There is no doubting the brilliance of Florence Nightingale's ideas. But the reason those ideas continue to resonate today is that she had the political savvy to get her ideas to the right people. For example, when Nightingale was commissioned to write a report on the future of St. Thomas Hospital in London—and she recommended that the venerable institution be torn down and rebuilt from scratch—she ensured her efforts would not gather dust on the shelf by preparing a single copy of the report to be sent to the Prince Consort, the hospital's most powerful leader. Nightingale was not only the first nursing leader, she was the profession's first skilled lobbyist.

One of the greatest challenges for the profession of nursing today is maintaining that tradition of excellent leadership, and of skilled communicators. That is the priority of Ginette Lemire

Rodger. She already has an impressive list of achievements as an academic, entrepreneur, and administrator. Lemire Rodger has also dabbled in politics, as a candidate for the federal Liberals. Now she is taking on a new, double challenge, as head nurse at the newly amalgamated Ottawa Hospital and as president of the Canadian Nurses Association. It is an intriguing combination, one that will keep her on the front lines and in the backrooms simultaneously, and virtually guarantee that nursing's profile will be raised several notches in the years to come.

Many of the nurses I talked to during the research for *Critical Care* spoke, almost wistfully, of how powerful nurses could be in Canada, if only they were united. With a quarter of a million registered nurses in Canada, the potential for influence is there. But it is untapped potential.

Shortages—the fact that nurses will be in demand after decades of being taken for granted—open the door to unleashing that potential. It is fitting that, as we enter the twenty-first century, the country's largest nursing organization has, at its helm, a woman who is truly a politician at heart, and a good one at that. Lemire Rodger understands power, as Nightingale did, and how to wield it responsibly. When nurses across Canada understand their strength, individual and collective, as well as she does, it will be a sight to behold. And the greatest beneficiaries will be consumers of health-care services.

Eyewitness to History—Élisabeth Carrier

Élisabeth Carrier's curriculum vitae reads like an atlas of misery: the killing fields of Cambodia; the slaughterhouse of Rwanda; the savage Afghan-Russian war; Iraq during the Persian Gulf war; civil war in Lebanon and Angola; ethnic slaughter in Croatia; refugee crises in Cameroon and Uganda; and civil unrest, starvation, and epidemics in Senegal, Chad, Kenya, the Republic of Georgia, and East Timor.

For a quarter of a century, the Red Cross nurse has travelled to the world's hot spots to minister to the sick and to promote human rights on behalf of the humanitarian organization. In the process, Carrier has been kidnapped by bandits, had her Jeep raked by gunfire, taken cover from shelling, narrowly averted drowning, been felled by disease, and witnessed untold horrors.

But she has always gone back for more. "After all this time, it's become a need, a calling," she says. "When I hear about a conflict, I just have to go—and I like it hot."

Carrier is soft-spoken, almost shy about her accomplishments. To get a true taste of Carrier's adventures, you have to read her book, titled *Entre le rire et les larmes* (*Between the Laughter and the Tears*). Even then she plays down the story, saying her experiences are not that different from those of many international-aid workers. "If there's one thing I must insist on, it's that I'm not the Mother Teresa of Quebec. It's nothing like that. The truth is that I'm privileged to have been an eyewitness to history," Carrier says.

She studied in Quebec City, but never practised in a hospital. Right after graduation in 1973, longing for adventure, the newly minted nurse headed to Northern Ontario to work in Attawapiskat, a desperately poor Cree village. From there, she headed even farther north, to another nursing station, in Kangiqsujuliak, an Inuit village of only 250 residents in subarctic Quebec. As a child, Carrier was entranced by the tales of a missionary uncle, and dreamed of Africa. The northern experience, with its epidemics of infectious disease, venereal diseases, and poverty, was a good primer.

Carrier's first stop abroad was in Gossas, Senegal, a remote part of the country where *kwashiorkor*, a form of malnutrition caused by severe protein deficiency, was rampant. She and the other nurses vaccinated tens of thousands of children, and established the region's first pharmacy, one stocked with drugs that cost only pennies but saved countless lives.

In 1979, Carrier was hired on a three-month contract by the Canadian Red Cross Society to be part of a medical team working in a refugee camp near the infamous Cambodian killing fields. She planned to return to university, but, just before classes began, an offer came to return to Africa. The battle on the Chad–Cameroon border was an ugly one, with bombs falling even on the refugee camp, and massive displacements of people. Carrier's work was largely dealing with infectious diseases that spread in the camps. "I'm not the nurse who treats the wounded coming back from battle. I'm the one dealing with everyone else affected by a conflict," she explains.

An average mission for Carrier lasted about six months because the stress of staying longer was too great. After all, the Red Cross is a charity that prides itself on working everywhere, even places that other international-aid groups consider too dangerous. Between missions, Carrier travelled to other, more comfortable parts of the world, but she would soon answer the siren call anew. Work took her from country to country, from hot spot to hot spot, and she soon became "not so much a citizen of the world as a citizen of nowhere." She also moved further away from traditional nursing, and increasingly into development and human-rights work. In Uganda, she found herself overseeing bridge repairs, rounding up crews to work in exchange for food.

While the work can be hard, and lonely, Carrier says she cannot imagine anything more rewarding. "The most inspiring thing is to be at the head of the convoy bringing food to starving people. You are, literally, saving their lives. There is such satisfaction knowing that you are making such a difference," she says. Like nursing, she adds, international-aid work "is not about sacrifice and courage, it's about discovery and joy."

In 1988, Carrier attempted to settle down again, but visits to hospitals in Quebec where she had applied to work left her convinced she could never adapt to institutional life. "The idea of working in an antiseptic, structured environment frightened me a lot more than running from bombs and struggling to find the most basic supplies," she says.

A call soon came for Carrier to join a mission in Afghanistan, and new challenges. There she had to deal with victims of a war where landmines—and blown-off limbs—were commonplace, and with an Islamic regime so zealous that it was virtually impossible to get even rubbing alcohol for medical purposes. Little did she know it would grow far worse on subsequent visits.

"Afghanistan is the country in the world that makes me saddest. When you know what women are going through under the Taliban regime, that, on the eve of the twenty-first century, women can be reduced to virtual slaves without the world crying out in anger, that is painful. It almost forces you to continue," Carrier says.

The time she came closest to quitting was December 17, 1996, one of the darkest days in Red Cross history. Canadian nurse Nancy Malloy was shot to death, along with five other workers, as they slept in a hospital dormitory in Chechnya. The slaughter shocked the world because it sent a message that the old rules were no longer being respected, that nurses and aid workers no longer had immunity, but could be targets in war zones. Malloy's killing hit Carrier hard for another reason.

"I was supposed to be there in Nancy's place. I was her replacement, but, at the last minute I was unable to go to Chechnya," she recalls, her voice dropping to a whisper. "All the women who didn't lock their doors that night were killed. Every day I ask myself, 'Would I have locked mine?' It's haunting." (Both Malloy and Carrier have received nursing's highest honour, the Florence Nightingale Medal.)

"Haunting" is also the word she uses to describe prisoner-of-war camps in Croatia. In the Balkans, Carrier was elevated to the status of International Red Cross delegate, verifying the conditions of prisoners of war and respect for the Geneva Convention. (There are only seventy-two such delegates worldwide.) "I met prisoners of war who could have been my father. They wept in my arms, pleading for their lives. It was horrible. It was horrible because it's so much like home, and look what happened there," she says.

Most recently, Carrier has returned to her nursing roots, tackling infectious-disease outbreaks, such as the epidemic of tuberculosis in the breakaway republics of the former Soviet Union. But she knows her days as an aid worker are numbered. The cumulative emotional strain is taking its toll, and the nurse is plagued with chronic backaches, the result of too much time spent in Jeeps, driving in conditions that are less than ideal, and too much heavy lifting.

Despite her decades abroad, home remains Saint-Étienne-de-Beaumont, a village just east of Quebec City on the shores of the St. Lawrence River, where, between missions, she operates a bed and breakfast, her harbour of peace in a world gone mad. Having re-established her base, she hopes to do what many nurses do at age 50: retire to a new line of work. She has already begun consulting in the international-aid field, and plans to spend time urging young nurses to follow in her footsteps.

Carrier says that, because so many health issues are intertwined with human-rights ones, there is a lot of room for nurses with a social conscience in non-governmental agencies. She stresses that, despite her spine-tingling tales, there are many uplifting times in the humanitarian field, and even many laughs. But she is determined to recruit younger workers because there are still too many failures, too many tears, and too few nurses lending a helping hand across international borders.

"I would like to say that I'm optimistic about the state of the world today, but, unfortunately, we are not lacking for work in my field. The world is still very much lacking in humanity. And if there is something that nurses can offer, in addition to their practical skills, it is compassion and kindness."

Sister of Charity—Rose Reynolds Nakatsuru

Brigida Reynolds was a nurse in England during the Second World War, coming to Canada as a war bride. She raised six children and did not return to work until her husband fell gravely ill and was unable to work—and then, because her nursing credentials had lapsed, she was a homemaker. Their daughter Rose was only eight when her father became paralysed and bed-ridden, and she learned caregiving skills beyond her years. The girl was fascinated by nursing, but felt she had done her time at home, and instead pursued an interest in the arts and business.

By 1993, Rose Reynolds Nakatsuru was working in investor relations at a large mining company, making a good living, but unsatisfied. So, at age 32, the Vancouver business woman decided, as had her mother before her, to become a nurse. Five years later, juggling family, work, and studies, full-time and part-time, she ended up with a degree.* But instead of taking a job at a hospital, where they are clamouring for new graduates, Reynolds used her nursing education to land a job at Canada's largest charitable foundation, the Vancouver Foundation.

Today, she is program director of the B.C. Medical Services Foundation,† a charity that doles out more than $1 million a year in grants for nursing research, medical research, and health promotion. The research money goes principally to university-based professors, while the health-promotion money tends to go to community groups.

Reynolds's job is to steer applicants through the process. She will provide them with guidelines, and ask for the idea to be explained in a letter of intent. If the project fits into the designated funding categories, she then invites a formal application, and provides technical assistance. The nurse will next assess in the field to determine if the applicant has the basic capacity to carry out the project, then, after reviewing all the material (in conjunction with a committee of experts), prepare a presentation and recommendation to the charity's board. The funding ranges from $1,000 bursaries up to $50,000 research grants.

For example, a large grant was given to researchers trying to determine the effectiveness of Osteofit, a community-based exercise program for post-menopausal women. In another instance, the B.C. Schizophrenia Society wanted to offer an education program in high schools, so the foundation underwrote the cost of

---

* The median age of nursing school graduates in Canada is 32.
† It was created in 1968 when the B.C. Medical Services Association wound down and had substantial funds left over. The endowment is administered by the Vancouver Foundation, which has almost $600 million in assets and itself gives out more than $25 million in grants annually.

a video and education kit for teenagers. Similarly, nurses and doctors at B.C. Children's Hospital who were concerned with antibiotic resistance got a small grant to draft an educational packet and launch a public-awareness campaign.

Reynolds delivers the good news—and the bad news to the unsuccessful—and does follow-up work to ensure the projects are carried out as proposed. She also sits on committees of the Vancouver Foundation, and assists with donor-recognition work. (Neither B.C. Meds nor the Vancouver Foundation does any fundraising, but, with their well-established reputation in the community, they attract a lot of donations, mostly from estates.)

Her nursing background has proved valuable because a lot of proposals are quite technical. She tries to look at the big picture, to determine how proposed research fits in to what's going on in the larger field of health care. It's a combination that many nurses know well: the medical and technical expertise, on the one hand, and, on the other, an awareness of what's going on in the community to be able to do their work in context.

Reynolds is the first nurse to hold the program director's job at B.C. Meds, and one result has been a lot more applications from community groups who had good ideas but were intimidated by the bureaucratic process. "I think people look to nurses as people who are nurturing and non-threatening. Whether you are giving them a needle or assisting them with paperwork, they trust that a nurse is going to help them in some way," she says.

Reynolds's interest was initially in community health, and she found herself doing practicums in a few groups that happened to get funding from the Vancouver Foundation. She decided to find out more about the group and, in doing so, landed a part-time receptionist's job at the charity, one that helped her make ends meet while studying.

Because of her nursing background and her interest in community health, Reynolds was asked to participate in a major research project sponsored by the Vancouver Foundation, called the Social Reconnaissance Project. Then, right around graduation time, the position at B.C. Meds opened up. "Some people think I'm not using my education appropriately, but I disagree," she says.

The job at B.C. Meds is three days a week, which also allows her time to do other kinds of nursing. To keep her licence as a practising nurse, she volunteers at a summer camp, and works several days a month at Healthy Beginnings, a prenatal community-health initiative sponsored by the foundation. Reynolds loves the flexibility, and sees herself following all kinds of paths—many that she cannot even envisage today—throughout her career.

"These days, you have to think about nursing in a different way. Why should we limit ourselves to the bedside, or to working our whole lives at one place, when there are all these opportunities in the community, in the non-profit sector and the corporate world?"

Healing the World—Margaret Hilson

On June 30, 1999, Margaret Hilson took to the stage in the Caxton Room of the Queen Elizabeth II Conference Centre in London, England, to a thunderous ovation from more than 4,000 nurses, and made history. At the International Congress of Nurses convention, she was singled out among more than 3 million nurses worldwide for the first-ever International Achievement Award of the Florence Nightingale International Foundation, in recognition of more than three decades of tireless health-promotion work.

In her acceptance speech, Hilson, director of international programs at the Canadian Public Health Association, said that health-care systems around the world must give nurses more power, support, and recognition. And nurses, she said, cannot content themselves merely with medical practice. "The main message I want to leave with you is that, to really improve the health of people, nurses must be more than health providers, we must be political activists and agents of change," she stated.

Hilson also spoke much of pride: her pride in being a nurse, her pride in Canada's universal health-care system, and her pride in the work Canadians have done to bring primary health care to many of the world's poorest. "Canada is an international leader in health promotion, and it's a reputation that's merited," she says.

Hilson has done a lot to shape that reputation. She started her nursing career doing community health work for the Victorian Order of Nurses (VON) in Cape Breton. Her two-year stint in one of Canada's poorest regions was her repayment to the VON for a bursary that put her through nursing school. The experience profoundly changed her view of health care and the role of nurses. Impassioned and adventurous, she joined Canadian University Services Overseas (as it was then known, or CUSO) and, in 1968, went to rural India. She has been involved in the field ever since, travelling and caring for patients all over Africa, Asia, and South America.

In the early days, Hilson was teaching family health and reproductive health to women who did not have access even to primary health care. "It was pretty basic. Nurses taught other women to teach. We would figure out the ten major health problems people have with their kids and teach them simple ways to prevent them," she says. After five years in India, she came back to Canada, to train other CUSO cooperants for overseas work, and got involved in policy development for the first time.

That interest in policy formulation would lead Hilson down a more radical path, to the political hotbeds of Latin America during the turbulent 1970s. In countries such as Nicaragua and Guatemala, the nurse worked with women's peasant farmers' organizations to develop village health programs and with gold miners' unions in assessing occupational-health-and-safety issues.

But the watershed event in her career was the 1978 Alma-Ata conference, where the United Nations set a goal of health for all by the year 2000. For the first time, churches, non-governmental agencies, and community-based nurses (notably Dame Nita Barrow)* had a major influence and that changed the face and the priorities

---

* An outspoken and articulate human-rights activist, Dame Nita Barrow started her career as a nurse in Barbados and rose to become a UN ambassador. She died in 1995.

of powerful agencies such as UNICEF and the World Health Organization. "The Alma-Ata declaration was a critical document, a human-rights manifesto that changed the world.* Now, we haven't been entirely successful in reaching the goal set out there—health for all in the twenty-first century—and that's sad, but there is not a country in the world today that does not have primary health care. It's not the same world as when I began," Hilson comments.

Around the world, it is nurses who deliver primary health care and, despite incredible odds, they are building paths to wellness, one child at a time. There are many countries where there is only one physician per 100,000 residents. Nurses do everything: prevention, education, treatment. Their most important role is health promotion, helping arm the next generation with the most powerful weapon in the health-care arsenal: knowledge.

Since joining the Canadian Public Health Association in 1985, where she now heads an interdisciplinary team of eleven nurses, doctors, environmentalists, and agronomists, Hilson has been trying to create and support projects that promote this basic knowledge. This is important because health is essential to the alleviation of poverty, and even to peace. "Health is an excellent entry point for people who want to change the world. Health is neutral, something that everyone, regardless of ideology, wants to promote. Regardless of their disagreements, people will agree immunizing children is a good thing. For example, at the height of war in El Salvador there was an immunization ceasefire. And, today, health is the issue that keeps Palestine and Israel at the table," she explains.

At this stage in her career, Hilson uses her expertise and renown to influence policy, and to help shape the next generation of caregiving. She sits on committees of the World Health Organization. She is an adviser to the minister of Foreign Affairs. She prods other health and welfare organizations to add or expand the international component of their activities. She lobbies the Canadian

* The International Conference on Primary Health Care, held in Alma-Ata, Soviet Union, in 1978, was among the first to link health and human rights.

International Development Agency (CIDA) not only for specific program funding, but for fundamental changes in their funding philosophy. "CIDA policy is that 25 per cent of money has to go to basic human needs. That's not enough. It should be 50 or 60 per cent," Hilson says bluntly.

She also spends a lot of her time sitting down with young health professionals, urging them to expand their horizons and to help maintain Canada's cherished position as a leader in health promotion. "I feel a tremendous obligation to get younger people interested, to get them excited about the big world of health care out there." Hilson says. A nurse today could probably not fashion a career like hers because one of the achievements of NGOs has been to help develop cadres of local health professionals. Still, there are many development groups that have important health-promotion components to their work, and even groups like Nobel Prize–winner Médecins Sans Frontières (Doctors Without Borders), where nurses are always in great demand.

The Canadian Public Health Association (CPHA) itself has an overseas office in Zimbabwe. One of its best-known projects is the Southern Africa AIDS Training Program, a mentoring program that focuses on the social impacts of the epidemic disease. The CPHA has developed programs to help villages take care of huge numbers of orphans, others to help disinherited widows fight to win legislative changes, and still more to teach family members to deliver basic home care and palliative care.

Hilson speaks eloquently about the ravages of AIDS on the African continent, but says we cannot allow them to overshadow all other positive realizations. "If you discount AIDS, the health of Africans has improved remarkably. Fewer children die, fewer mothers die, life expectancy is up, more people have water, and more people have health care. Even the AIDS epidemic has a positive side, if I can say it that way. It is changing the face of Africa, forcing fundamental societal changes that will forever improve health promotion and the delivery of health care. AIDS will pass, but these changes will be lasting."

Nursing and development work abroad have made Hilson very aware of the social and medical costs of poverty. Hilson says health promotion is something Canadians take too much for granted, smugly ignoring prevention because they are convinced that technology can save them. She believes the wisest course is to spend more on health promotion not only at home, but overseas, because epidemics now travel at the speed of jet aircraft. And having an international perspective makes her appreciate our universal medicare system. "Sure, it has some problems, but I'm astounded that Canadians don't have a lot more pride in the system, that they don't fight for it a lot more vigorously. Maybe they should travel more, because I can't think of any country in the world that wouldn't love this health-care system, warts and all. It's really a model for the world, but we have done a terrible job of marketing it, of promoting the public system."

Hilson says the greatest thing about being a nurse is that it is the most recognizable and most admired profession on the planet. "Being a nurse has never been an obstacle, it has always been a door opener." Even though she has not done hands-on care for many years—calling herself "de-skilled"—Hilson says her background as a nurse has always been indispensable. "It's influenced everything I've done and, to this day, there's nothing more thrilling for me than going to a clinic, say in Malawi, and watching a nurse fill in a growth chart. That nursing background keeps you grounded, it keeps you aware of what's really important in the world."

In fact, Hilson is at odds with the Ontario College of Nurses, the licensing body, which has some doubts about her still being classified as a nurse. "Of course, I still think what I do is nursing. As the world changes, they're going to have to get their heads around things like this, and realize the fundamental importance of health promotion," she says. While she may no longer have the skills to save the life of an individual, Hilson has developed something far more precious: the ability to reshape entire systems, to influence the way health care is delivered around the world today and for many years to come.

The Corporate Caregiver—Mary Ferguson-Paré

Mary Ferguson-Paré is trying to describe her typical workday. She hasn't yet finished outlining the early-morning meetings that take her up to a normal breakfast time when she interrupts herself: "Let's face it, I spend my life in meetings. More meetings than you could ever imagine." As vice-president of professional affairs, human resources, and organizational development at Vancouver Hospital and Health Sciences Centre, she has a finger in virtually every aspect of the vast institution's operations.*

"It's wild. But my clinical background is in psychiatric nursing so, jokingly, I say that's what allows me to do this job. It's what makes me a good administrator," Ferguson-Paré says.

A growing number of nurses are climbing the executive ladder, ever so slowly, and changing institutions. But, paradoxically, the ascent of nurses into the inner sanctum of administration is coming at a time of unprecedented disdain (and sometimes open attacks) on the nursing profession. For those who, like Ferguson-Paré, retain a passion for nursing, who believe the role of nurses should be expanded not contracted, that creates daily dilemmas.

"With full respect, I have to say that people in positions of power like mine often find themselves in politically compromising positions that are not good for nursing. Unfortunately, many nurses have taken an ecumenical approach when they get to the management level. That disappoints nurses who count on them to carry the day on every issue. But when you're in a position like mine, you have to decide: 'What hill am I going to die on?'" she says, demonstrating her uncommon frankness.

One of Ferguson-Paré's principal interests, and the subject of much of her research, is building nursing leadership by promoting

* Ferguson-Paré has since become vice-president of nursing at Baycrest Centre for Geriatric Care, where she is responsible for nursing practice, education, and research, as well as operations. It is a similar position but with a stricter focus on nursing. Baycrest is a smaller institution but has a reputation for innovation and cutting-edge research.

greater autonomy in practice. She is disturbed by the widespread elimination of the head-nurse position, the woman so many nurses looked to for guidance and support.

She is also troubled by the treatment of nurse-managers in crunch times. "When they started restructuring in Ontario, the nurses in positions like mine spoke out forcefully against compromising care, against the layoff of nurses. The result is that many of their positions were eliminated. Nurses often criticize their colleagues who are managers but they have to realize that, at the corporate level, you are very vulnerable, and that sometimes silences voices that should be heard," she asserts.

Ferguson-Paré is not the type to be silenced. She has muscled her way to the top with a combination of impressive academic credentials—including a master's in public health administration, and a master's and doctorate in organizational development*— and formidable management skills. As such, she is a headhunter's dream, but has spurned repeated lucrative offers from big business. "There's an inherent value in my work that wouldn't be there in widget production. I just wouldn't be excited creating widgets the way I am delivering health care."

Despite her fancy title and her power as a key administrator of a hospital with 2,000 beds, five sites, 9,000 employees, and an annual budget of $525 million, Ferguson-Paré thinks of herself as, first and foremost, a nurse. "I'm not at the bedside anymore, but everything I do creates the context for direct care delivery. I'm the support staff, the facilitator, for all the really good stuff that happens out there in the hospital—like nursing," she says.

She wishes that all nurses could, like her, have the opportunity to be creative in their jobs, to experience the infinite opportunities that nursing creates. But as the manager responsible for human resources and organizational structures, Ferguson-Paré feels that many nurses are being held back by labour agreements. While

* She credits her mother, a nurse, for her success. It was her mother who, in the 1960s, insisted that Ferguson-Paré get a bachelor's in nursing, predicting it would be mandatory in the future.

unions helped nurses attain decent wage levels, she feels they have become the worst enemy of dynamic nurses who are looking for challenges. In particular, labour contracts fail to take into account the growing specialization of nurses. "One of the most stultifying areas of nursing is that collective agreements state that a nurse is a nurse is a nurse. That's absolute nonsense. It's inappropriate to say that nurses are interchangeable. I believe you should be able to pay and promote based on expertise and performance, but seniority reigns," she says.

At Vancouver Hospital, Ferguson-Paré dedicated much of her time and effort to developing and implementing a model for patient-centred care, one that has expanded professional practice and consumer feedback as central components. While creating organizational infrastructures sounds like horribly tedious and technical work, it is essential to the future of the health-care system itself, she stresses. She understands the business of health care and the importance of creating, from a corporate perspective, good care. Her goal is to create an environment where nurses and patients can thrive.

Ferguson-Paré notes that much of the change in the health-care system is being driven by baby boomers, who have a more consumer-oriented approach than previous generations. "Partnership is a big deal for health consumers today. Boomers do not want to be passive patients. They want to know how they can contribute to their wellness and health. They don't want to wait to fall ill, then get treated for some disease. They want to be dealt with as whole people, in the context of their job, family, and community," she says. This is precisely the type of care that, when they can define their practice, nurses provide. Ferguson-Paré knows that this represents the future of what is being sought by consumers.

Yet, the system, with few exceptions, prevents nurses from practising to the best of their abilities. Work is designed around tasks instead of around patient needs. "We have systematically taken away the piece that is the heart, the essence of nursing—patient care. When nurses say: 'We don't have time to spend with our patients anymore' there is something seriously wrong. How can you get job satisfaction—and how can patients get proper care—when you are systematically deprived of the ability to do the core of your work?" Ferguson-Paré asks.

As the manager responsible for human resources—notably the recruitment and retention of nurses—she spends a lot of her time thinking about nursing shortages. "It is literally the corporate priority of this hospital, and many other health-care institutions. The president tells me regularly to drop everything and dedicate myself to the issue of shortages because he is worried about not being able to provide service," Ferguson-Paré says. "We are already closing beds because of shortages, and this is only the beginning of what could be a long, dark slide."

An expert in so-called magnet hospitals—those that have a reputation as good places to practise nursing and which, as a result, do not have shortages—Ferguson-Paré believes the basis of a solution lies in creating attractive, supportive workplaces for nurses. Administrators at Vancouver Hospital make it a point to meet every single graduate of nursing schools in B.C. to make a pitch. "I'm promising them the world," says Ferguson-Paré, and she wishes she could offer more. "In the U.S., they come up with $10,000 bonuses, housing, education grants, different shifts. They have a flexibility that we don't have in a highly unionized public sector," she says.

As a senior manager, Ferguson-Paré is particularly frustrated by the fact that today's shortages were entirely predictable and largely preventable. Hospitals have known since the early 1980s what was required to keep nurses happy, but they have not systematically restructured in a manner to prevent shortages. Ferguson-Paré believes the underlying reason is that nurses don't have enough power and control.

"Nursing seems to be the only profession, and certainly the only health profession, where everyone and their dog feels they should have a say. I can't think of another discipline that doesn't have command of itself, that is at the mercy of others," Ferguson-Paré complains. "Because nursing is predominantly women and about caring, it has been meddled with since time immemorial by policy-makers. The power of nursing comes from a collective voice, and we have to rediscover that collective voice."

The Siren Song—Linda Beechinor

In 1985, Linda Beechinor was at wit's end. Since graduating from St. Paul's Hospital in Vancouver more than a decade earlier, she had worked at a number of surgical and obstetrical nursing jobs in B.C. and Alberta but, like so many of her counterparts, was unable to secure a permanent position. She had turned to teaching, but that, too, seemed like a dead end because, with few job prospects, students weren't exactly flocking to nursing schools.

Beechinor heard that prospects were a lot better in the United States. Looking for adventure—and good weather—she set her sights on Hawaii. First, she called around to hospitals. Encouraged, she travelled to Honolulu. There she found chronic shortages and hospitals tripping over each other to hire her, given the years of experience she had accumulated in surgery and academia. But Beechinor was also surprised to learn that employers' enthusiasm was not coupled with knowledge. "They wanted to hire me, but didn't have a clue about logistics. I had to arrange my own visa, find a place to stay, and adapt to a new system all on my own," Beechinor says.

In other words, not only were hospitals not recruiting, they had no idea how to do so. Used to reinventing herself in the scramble for work in Canada, Beechinor saw an opportunity—and doubly so when she realized that there were hundreds of nurses from around Asia already living in nurse-poor Hawaii but unable to work because they had not passed their U.S. exams.

"I had this background in education, so I decided to develop a course and market it to schools of nursing in Asia. They could upgrade and modify their teaching, and graduates would be ready to pass the U.S. exams," Beechinor says. The course was an instant hit, and that created a new opportunity. "Once students took the course, they were all asking me for jobs. They looked at me as the expert. So I approached local employers and said I could bring them a steady supply of nurses who passed the U.S. exams. They were thrilled, and things kind of took off from there," she says.

Meanwhile, like all nurses who head off abroad, she was getting inquiries from friends and colleagues back in Canada. Her mother—as all mothers do—worried that her daughter was lonely so far from home. So, when Beechinor was coming home for a visit, her mother took out a small ad in the *Vancouver Sun*, urging nurses who were looking for work in Hawaii to contact her. "It was quite a surprise because the phone rang off the hook for days and drove the family absolutely crazy," Beechinor recalls with a laugh.

Since then, she has recruited more than 400 Canadian nurses to Hawaii, making them a significant minority among the state's nursing workforce of 6,000. "They love Canadian nurses here. The Canadian nursing-education system is very well thought of, so the employers know they're going to get top-notch nurses. Canadian nurses—maybe because of our medicare system—are also very active, very passionate about their work. That means they are very visible, and lots of them move into management jobs," she says. "For us, nursing isn't just a job, it's a career."

Beechinor, for example, has a nursing life that would make most blanch. She operates a full-time recruiting business. She runs her own clinical practice (Hawaii has nurse-practitioners whose role is similar to that of family physicians in Canada), a mobile clinic offering free medical help to uninsured immigrants. She teaches full-time in the nursing faculty at the University of Hawaii. And she is the former president of the Association of Hawaiian Nurses.

As her experience demonstrates, Beechinor says, Canadian nurses fit in socially and culturally. They feel a lot more comfortable in Hawaii than most mainland U.S. nurses. Honolulu, like Vancouver and Toronto, is a cosmopolitan, multicultural city, without the segregation you see in most big U.S. cities. "Canadians are a lot like Hawaiians in their temperament. They're quiet and observant, not loud and pushy like many Americans," the recruiter says. Hawaii also has something that distinguishes it greatly from most mainland states—universal health insurance. (In Hawaii, employers are obliged to provide health insurance to all workers and their families. The state has virtually no unemployment, so very few are uninsured.)

If there is one thing that turns off nurses who have gone to work in the United States, it is the cost to patients, the horror of demanding to get a patient's insurance details or credit card before they can be treated. "But it's a lot more like Canada here. Hospitals don't really turn people away," Beechinor says. Another shock to many nurses who emigrate is the cost of liability insurance, a necessary protection from a litigious public. But Hawaii's system is centralized, meaning nurses pay only $78 annually for $3 million in insurance coverage.

The state is also highly unionized (including 95 per cent of nurses), meaning wages are high and benefits are excellent. But the real attraction is job security. An experienced nurse, particularly one with a specialty that's in demand (critical care, dialysis, pediatric, ICU) can readily get excellent-paying, permanent employment.

Beechinor has delivered on that promise so many times that she does not even attend job fairs or advertise;* she depends on word of mouth. And she places more than one in twenty of the nurses who contact her in jobs, a rate that is many times higher than that achieved by most recruiters. But Beechinor is obviously not an average recruiter. She denounces job fairs as "degrading meat markets," and says the image of recruitment firms as sleazy headhunters is well deserved. "Among working nurses, the image of recruiters is very negative, and that's quite accurate. But just look who's doing it: It's big business who are out for business, not out there to protect the interests of nurses."

Beechinor, like all recruiters, works for the employer. She is a

---

* With one exception. In each edition of *Canadian Nurse* she runs a classified ad that reads simply: "Hawaii needs experienced nurses. Full-time positions with benefits. Families welcome." Her phone number follows.

consultant who gets paid for delivering a needed employee. But, unlike most recruiters, she charges a set fee and will not take any money from nurses themselves (such as a percentage of salary or a recruitment fee).

"When I get called a 'headhunter,' I just laugh. I'm not sitting in some office tower in Chicago looking for warm bodies to make money from. The main reason I got into this business is because I thought recruitment should be a nursing function. There are opportunities out there for nurses, but they should hear about them from a nursing perspective, from someone who can vouch for the employers personally," she says.

Beechinor knows that, in some circles, she is vilified as a traitor, as someone who is contributing to the nursing brain drain to the United States. But she makes no apologies. "I worked in Canada for fifteen years before coming here. I never would have left if the working conditions were better, and that's true of everyone I've recruited. I have a lot of nurses who call me these days who have been casual employees for ten years, who juggle shifts in three or four hospitals, and they're sick of it. The way nurses are treated in Canada is appalling. You can pretend they come here for the weather or the lower taxes, but that's not true." When Beechinor promises a full-time job with full benefits, permanent, nurses are delighted. "They would do the same thing if you gave them those opportunities in Winnipeg or Vancouver or Moose Jaw," Beechinor says.

The recruiter is well aware of the projected shortages in Canada. In fact, she believes they will be worse than predicted, not due to sheer numbers, but because the experienced, specialized nurses are increasingly those who are leaving the country. It used to be that young, unmarried women came to Hawaii to work. They were looking for adventure, and could take off for a year or two. Today, there is no shortage of young graduates. But Beechinor is increasingly recruiting older, experienced nurses (almost all with families) because, when they make a commitment to come, it's usually for the long term, and employers like that.

While Beechinor loves Canada's public-health system, the

As she climbed the management ladder, Shamian also studied, earning a nursing degree at Concordia University, a master's in public health at York University, and a doctorate in nursing administration at Case-Western University in Cleveland. She also served on the College of Nurses of Ontario, as a board member of the Canadian Nurses Association, and as president of the Registered Nurses Association of Ontario (RNAO).

"Throughout my career, I have always been guided by one fundamental question: 'How can you make a difference?'" she says. Today, Shamian believes the answer to that question is by applying all her experience to policy work. In particular, she would like to reverse a troubling trend that she has seen develop over the years—and in an accelerated fashion since cutbacks began in earnest in 1993—namely, the deterioration of work conditions for nurses. She knows that there are a lot of issues that need to be addressed in a systematic fashion at a policy level: injuries (Shamian had her bedside career cut short at age 26 by a serious back injury),* casualization, shift work, nurse–patient ratios, to name a few. What is clear to her is that we cannot expect nurses to carry the primary burden of downsizing. If we continue to do so, patients will be put at risk.

One of the frustrations she feels is that everyone agrees that the health-care system needs more, not fewer, nurses, but no concerted effort is being made to see that it happens. "The CEOs will tell you that, the governments will tell you that, the unions will tell you that, the nurses themselves will tell you that, and, above all, the patients will tell you that. So where is the action?" she wonders.

Shamian, however, remains optimistic that the big issues will be not only addressed, but resolved, in the relatively near future. The reason is that nurses are learning to speak out at a time when consumers are becoming more demanding, creating a "dynamic synergy" that will force the hand of politicians.

* Research has shown that about 40 per cent of nurses suffer from chronic back pain due to injuries sustained on the job.

recruiter believes there are some important lessons the state-run system should learn from private and non-profit enteprise in the United States. (Most of Hawaii's hospitals are actually non-profit institutions, but they are quite competitive.) "The hospitals here are businesses, but that's not all bad. In fact, for nurses, it's quite good. Hospitals have learned to not skimp on nursing care. That's their product: More than anything else, they sell nursing care. So nurses here are treated very well," she says.

Rather than complain about nurses taking jobs in the United States, Beechinor says, employers in Canada should study the reasons for their departure, and learn from them. "It's been clear for twenty years why nurses leave Canada. It's work conditions. Period. It's not anything else. If work conditions were good at home, if nurses were respected the way they are here, I wouldn't recruit a soul."

The Head Nurse—Judith Shamian

"You only have to look into the eyes of nurses to see the price they are paying. That personal struggle to maintain quality care is very real, it's very painful, and it should worry each and every one of us, because we will all need the health-care system some day," says Judith Shamian, leaning forward and tapping her pencil forcefully on a notepad for emphasis.

"There is not, in government today, at a policy level, a clear understanding of just how hard it is to be a nurse. I think it is ethically irresponsible for that situation to continue. It is intolerable," she says.

Blunt, forceful talk is Shamian's trademark. And despite protestations that she has mellowed, the veteran nurse does not shy away from expressing her opinions, even though she has herself joined the federal bureaucracy. As executive director of nursing policy at Health Canada, she became the country's *de facto* head nurse when she took up her post in the fall of 1999.

Shamian's role is twofold. First and foremost, she brings a nursing perspective to a broad range of policy decisions. Just a couple of weeks into the new job, she already had two large briefcases full of briefing material on a variety of current topics. Now, when policies are formulated on major health issues such as reproductive technologies, euthanasia, home care, pharmacare, and privatization, Shamian is an integral part of the internal debate. She does so from a senior position, one with direct access to the deputy minister, and even the minister, of Health.

"This role is exciting because I will be a very active member in describing and thinking through what the Canadian health-care system should look like in the future. This is the highest policy position one can reach in shaping this national treasure we call medicare, and it is long overdue that a nursing perspective be included," Shamian says. "At this level of decision making, people are looking for intellectual debate and strong opinions, and they're going to get both from me."

The second aspect of her job is to keep abreast of major issues within the nursing profession, and to serve as a facilitator among the various players in the health-care sector when there is a need to find solutions. Number one on her list, obviously, is shortages. With projections of shortfalls as severe as 113,000 within a decade, Shamian recognizes that there is much work to be done. But she also has no doubt about her goal.

"The health human-resource issue is a priority. The question is not merely how we will get through another cycle of shortages. We need a long-term perspective for resolving this problem. We need to change the system so this problem is not only resolved, but does not recur," she says.

As a long-time researcher, Shamian has as her starting point empirical data. "I like to make changes based on evidence, not on speculation. We need a good understanding of the reasons there are shortages before we can find lasting solutions. For example, I don't deny for a minute that there is a brain drain of nurses, but we have to find out Who? Why? and When? Once we empower ourselves with knowledge, we will be able to act decisively," she says.

Shamian showed the power of knowledge—and nursing—in her

previous position as vice-president of nursing at Toronto's Mount Sinai Hospital. When most other hospitals in North America were cutting nursing staff and replacing them with lesser-skilled nursing assistants, she not only maintained, but also bolstered, nursing staff. What her rigorously compiled data showed was that, once the costs of training and supervising less-skilled staff were factored in, cutting nurses would actually cost the hospital money. Today, Mount Sinai remains one of the few hospitals where all nursing staff are registered nurses.

Shamian is also fondly remembered at the hospital for her accessibility. She hosted monthly forums where nurses could give their feedback and suggestions, and always had time for one-on-one meetings. It is a philosophy she has carried over to Health Canada, a breath of fresh air in a notoriously secretive and inward-looking ministry. "My intention is to connect with multiple groups—unions, nursing associations, regulatory bodies, hospital administrators, community groups—and to do so wherever I can—conferences, roundtables, and other areas," she says. "And I think it's important for everyone, particularly the nursing groups, to realize that I'm not there to replace them. Their input and influence must continue, and I will be one more voice at the table t[o] complement that role."

Shamian's goal, admittedly a lofty one, is to do on a natio[nal] level what she has done in the hospital setting: to advocate [and] champion the role of the nurse. She feels that nurses need t[o be] valued not only in words, but in deeds.

Most of her career—professional, educational, and volunt[eer] has been dedicated to doing so. Shamian began her nursing [career] at Shaare-Zedek Hospital in Jerusalem, as an emergency [room] nurse during the 1973 war. She then worked as a com[munity] nurse on a kibbutz, acting as the sole health-care provid[er for a] community of 500. From there she jumped back to the [hospital] setting, serving a variety of staff nursing and managem[ent posi-]tions at Jewish General Hospital in Montreal, as directo[r of nurs-]ing research at Sunnybrook, then as vice-president at M[ount] recruiter believes there are some important lessons the state-run system should learn from private and non-profit enteprise in the United States. (Most of Hawaii's hospitals are actually non-profit institutions, but they are quite competitive.) "The hospitals here are businesses, but that's not all bad. In fact, for nurses, it's quite good. Hospitals have learned to not skimp on nursing care. That's their product: More than anything else, they sell nursing care. So nurses here are treated very well," she says.

Rather than complain about nurses taking jobs in the United States, Beechinor says, employers in Canada should study the reasons for their departure, and learn from them. "It's been clear for twenty years why nurses leave Canada. It's work conditions. Period. It's not anything else. If work conditions were good at home, if nurses were respected the way they are here, I wouldn't recruit a soul."

The Head Nurse—Judith Shamian

"You only have to look into the eyes of nurses to see the price they are paying. That personal struggle to maintain quality care is very real, it's very painful, and it should worry each and every one of us, because we will all need the health-care system some day," says Judith Shamian, leaning forward and tapping her pencil forcefully on a notepad for emphasis.

"There is not, in government today, at a policy level, a clear understanding of just how hard it is to be a nurse. I think it is ethically irresponsible for that situation to continue. It is intolerable," she says.

Blunt, forceful talk is Shamian's trademark. And despite protestations that she has mellowed, the veteran nurse does not shy away from expressing her opinions, even though she has herself joined the federal bureaucracy. As executive director of nursing policy at Health Canada, she became the country's *de facto* head nurse when she took up her post in the fall of 1999.

Shamian's role is twofold. First and foremost, she brings a nursing perspective to a broad range of policy decisions. Just a couple of weeks into the new job, she already had two large briefcases full of briefing material on a variety of current topics. Now, when policies are formulated on major health issues such as reproductive technologies, euthanasia, home care, pharmacare, and privatization, Shamian is an integral part of the internal debate. She does so from a senior position, one with direct access to the deputy minister, and even the minister, of Health.

"This role is exciting because I will be a very active member in describing and thinking through what the Canadian health-care system should look like in the future. This is the highest policy position one can reach in shaping this national treasure we call medicare, and it is long overdue that a nursing perspective be included," Shamian says. "At this level of decision making, people are looking for intellectual debate and strong opinions, and they're going to get both from me."

The second aspect of her job is to keep abreast of major issues within the nursing profession, and to serve as a facilitator among the various players in the health-care sector when there is a need to find solutions. Number one on her list, obviously, is shortages. With projections of shortfalls as severe as 113,000 within a decade, Shamian recognizes that there is much work to be done. But she also has no doubt about her goal.

"The health human-resource issue is a priority. The question is not merely how we will get through another cycle of shortages. We need a long-term perspective for resolving this problem. We need to change the system so this problem is not only resolved, but does not recur," she says.

As a long-time researcher, Shamian has as her starting point empirical data. "I like to make changes based on evidence, not on speculation. We need a good understanding of the reasons there are shortages before we can find lasting solutions. For example, I don't deny for a minute that there is a brain drain of nurses, but we have to find out Who? Why? and When? Once we empower ourselves with knowledge, we will be able to act decisively," she says.

Shamian showed the power of knowledge—and nursing—in her

previous position as vice-president of nursing at Toronto's Mount Sinai Hospital. When most other hospitals in North America were cutting nursing staff and replacing them with lesser-skilled nursing assistants, she not only maintained, but also bolstered, nursing staff. What her rigorously compiled data showed was that, once the costs of training and supervising less-skilled staff were factored in, cutting nurses would actually cost the hospital money. Today, Mount Sinai remains one of the few hospitals where all nursing staff are registered nurses.

Shamian is also fondly remembered at the hospital for her accessibility. She hosted monthly forums where nurses could give their feedback and suggestions, and always had time for one-on-one meetings. It is a philosophy she has carried over to Health Canada, a breath of fresh air in a notoriously secretive and inward-looking ministry. "My intention is to connect with multiple groups—unions, nursing associations, regulatory bodies, hospital administrators, community groups—and to do so wherever I can—conferences, roundtables, and other areas," she says. "And I think it's important for everyone, particularly the nursing groups, to realize that I'm not there to replace them. Their input and influence must continue, and I will be one more voice at the table to complement that role."

Shamian's goal, admittedly a lofty one, is to do on a national level what she has done in the hospital setting: to advocate and champion the role of the nurse. She feels that nurses need to be valued not only in words, but in deeds.

Most of her career—professional, educational, and volunteer—has been dedicated to doing so. Shamian began her nursing career at Shaare-Zedek Hospital in Jerusalem, as an emergency-room nurse during the 1973 war. She then worked as a community nurse on a kibbutz, acting as the sole health-care provider for a community of 500. From there she jumped back to the hospital setting, serving a variety of staff nursing and management functions at Jewish General Hospital in Montreal, as director of nursing research at Sunnybrook, then as vice-president at Mount Sinai.

As she climbed the management ladder, Shamian also studied, earning a nursing degree at Concordia University, a master's in public health at York University, and a doctorate in nursing administration at Case-Western University in Cleveland. She also served on the College of Nurses of Ontario, as a board member of the Canadian Nurses Association, and as president of the Registered Nurses Association of Ontario (RNAO).

"Throughout my career, I have always been guided by one fundamental question: 'How can you make a difference?'" she says. Today, Shamian believes the answer to that question is by applying all her experience to policy work. In particular, she would like to reverse a troubling trend that she has seen develop over the years—and in an accelerated fashion since cutbacks began in earnest in 1993—namely, the deterioration of work conditions for nurses. She knows that there are a lot of issues that need to be addressed in a systematic fashion at a policy level: injuries (Shamian had her bedside career cut short at age 26 by a serious back injury),* casualization, shift work, nurse–patient ratios, to name a few. What is clear to her is that we cannot expect nurses to carry the primary burden of downsizing. If we continue to do so, patients will be put at risk.

One of the frustrations she feels is that everyone agrees that the health-care system needs more, not fewer, nurses, but no concerted effort is being made to see that it happens. "The CEOs will tell you that, the governments will tell you that, the unions will tell you that, the nurses themselves will tell you that, and, above all, the patients will tell you that. So where is the action?" she wonders.

Shamian, however, remains optimistic that the big issues will be not only addressed, but resolved, in the relatively near future. The reason is that nurses are learning to speak out at a time when consumers are becoming more demanding, creating a "dynamic synergy" that will force the hand of politicians.

---

* Research has shown that about 40 per cent of nurses suffer from chronic back pain due to injuries sustained on the job.